D1566082

Table of Contents

Chapter 1: Physical Care Skills—Activities of Daily Living

As a certified nursing assistant, you will be responsible for assisting clients of all ages who are recovering from diseases, injuries, surgery, and procedures. For example, certified nursing assistants care for infants after they are born, for the elderly in their home or in a long-term care facility, and for clients of all ages in a hospital.

Dorothea Orem's Self-Care theory is a good framework to use in terms of self-care and the activities of daily living. This theory states that clients can, and want to, care for themselves as much as possible. The three types of nursing systems that Orem identifies are the supportive-educative (developmental), partly compensatory, and the wholly compensatory nursing systems.

The supportive-educative (developmental) nursing system aims to provide clients with the support, assistance, and care they need to continue their independent self-care. These patients may just need a reminder or a little help gathering supplies; however, they are able to perform their own independent self-care and activities of daily living.

The partly compensatory nursing system meets the self-care needs of clients who can perform some, but not all, self-care functions and activities of daily living. These patients may need, for example, some help getting out of bed and/or washing their back. The nursing assistant helps these patients by giving them as much independence as possible and helping only with those things patients cannot do on their own.

Lastly, the wholly compensatory nursing system provides all care to clients because they are unable to perform any self-care. Infants, very young children, and clients in a coma are examples of clients needing wholly compensatory nursing care. At this level, the nursing assistant provides all care in terms of bathing, hygiene, and other activities of daily living.

Nursing assistants care for some clients who can take care of personal care needs without any help; others may require only a little help, while still other clients need much help.

When the client is able to take care of personal care needs without any help, the nursing assistant does not need to do anything besides provide privacy and gather the items they need.

It is very important to encourage clients to perform self-care and be independent as much as possible. The patient's levels of self-esteem, dignity, sense of control, and quality of life increase when he/she is independent with activities of daily living.

Nursing assistants provide only necessary care for clients who are unable to perform some, or all, personal care needs because they are too young or old, too confused or disoriented, or too sick or physically disabled. The amount of help the nursing assistant provides depends on the individual client and his/her needs.

When helping the client with personal care needs, several things must be done:

- Wash your hands, put on gloves before any care is provided, and use standard precautions.

- Greet the client, introduce yourself with your full name and title (nursing assistant or certified nursing assistant), and tell the patient what you are going to do for and with him/her before you provide any care.

- Verify the client's identity including name, date of birth, and any other required verification items. All processes, including personal care, require verification of the client's identity. Failure to check the client's identity can lead to serious, and sometimes deadly, mistakes.

- Ensure the patient is safe at all times. Maintaining safety includes ensuring the water temperature in a bath or shower is safe and never leaving a client alone when he/she is very young, confused, or unable to safely bathe alone. Very little water is needed for an accidental drowning. You must also prevent falls by ensuring the floor is not wet or cluttered; by ensuring all safety bars, grab bars, and shower chairs are strong enough and safe enough to hold the client's weight; and, if giving a patient a bed bath, ensuring the bed is never left in a high position unless you are close by and monitoring the client.

- Be prepared. Have all supplies gathered and ready to use. For example, before the client enters the tub or shower, ensure the shampoo, soap, and towels are at arm's length from the shower or tub.

- Observe the patient while personal care is given. For example, observe and check his/her skin for any paleness, tears, sores, redness, or breakdown. Communicate with the client and observe his/her mental state. Is the client more or less confused than he/she was previously? Does the client know where he/she is? Does he/she know what day, month, and year it is? Does he/she have any fears or concerns? If any of your observations are NOT normal and/or NOT normal for the client, immediately report these findings and observations to the nurse.

- Allow the client to choose when he/she wants different personal care needs completed. For example, one client may prefer to bathe in the morning, while another client may choose to bathe in the afternoon.

- Feel the patient. Is he/she hot, cold, sweaty, or moist?

- Smell the patient. Does the patient have any unusual odors?

- Treat the client with respect, kindness, and dignity at all times. Make the client comfortable and enable him/her to enjoy the personal care aspects of his/her life.

HYGIENE

Bathing

Bathing is extremely beneficial to the client. Bathing cleans away all of the dirt, sweat, germs, adhesive, iodine, and blood that can dry up on the skin. Bathing makes the patient feel better, and it prevents infections and promotes good blood flow in the client's body.

Some clients are inclined to bathe only every other day, whereas other clients may choose to bathe several times a day, especially when they are incontinent of urine and/or stool. Some patients elect to bathe in the morning, while others choose afternoons or evenings. It is always the client's choice as to when and how often to bathe, as well as the type of bath, so always let the client choose and follow his/her individual choice.

In the healthcare setting, there are three different types of baths: complete bath, partial bath, and tub or shower bath.

A *compete bath* is a bath given entirely in the bed by the nursing assistant or other member of the healthcare team. A *partial bath* is a bath given in the bed, but unlike the complete bath, the healthcare worker assists the client with some aspects of the bath such as washing the back, towel drying the client, and/or washing the feet. A *tub or shower bath* is a bath that clients are able to take themselves; however, they may still need assistance getting in or out of the tub or shower, so it is important that the nursing assistant be available and present to help as needed.

Supervision is always necessary with tub and shower baths to prevent slips, falls, and even drowning. Respecting the client's privacy and treating the client with dignity and respect are also highly important. At times, privacy needs must be carefully balanced with safety needs.

With all types of baths, the water must be checked to ensure the correct temperature. The water temperature can vary, depending on the client's preferences, but it should never exceed 110° F. Hot water can be harmful and can even cause burns. Many facilities have temperature regulators either built into the tub or available for use. Another way to check the water temperature is with a bath thermometer. If none of these are available, check the water temperature on your wrist before the client bathes or enters the tub.

Before beginning the bathing process, collect all necessary supplies, including extra towels and washcloths, then wash your hands thoroughly and put on gloves. Always greet the client, verify his/her identity, and let him/her know what you are going to be doing. If there is any sign that the client does not want to bathe at that time, respect his/her wishes and report it to the nurse because the client's wishes must be heard and accommodated.

Below are the steps for a complete bath and a partial bath. The procedure for a partial bath depends on what the client can do without the nursing assistant's help.

- Completely remove the client's blankets and any other top sheets or coverings so they do not get wet. Towels should be placed under the areas being washed to protect the fitted bottom sheet from getting wet during the bath.

- Raise the client's bed to a height that is most comfortable and safe, in terms of body mechanics, for you to work. Ensure the side rail on the bed opposite of you is up and locked in place. Raise the head of the bed to a comfortable height for the client.

- Take off the client's clothing or gown completely, then cover the patient with a bath towel to provide comfort, warmth, and privacy.

- Each part of the client's body is washed, rinsed, dried, and then recovered with the bath towel or blanket.

- If a bath mitt is unavailable, the washcloth should be wrapped around your hand in a mitt-like fashion.

- Rinse off the mitt or washcloth completely after washing each part of the body.

- If the water gets cold or appears cloudy or too soapy, it should be changed. If you must leave the bedside for any reason, ensure the client is safe by lowering the bed to its lowest and safest height.

- Ensure that every area including the face, behind the ears, chest, back, arms, legs, hands, fingernails, perineal area, feet, etc. is washed, rinsed, and dried thoroughly. When you move from one side of the bed to the other, raise and lock the side rail opposite from the side of the bed on which you are working.

- Dress the client after the bath is done.

- Lower the bed and, if possible, soak the client's feet, wash the feet, and clean the toenails (with a nail brush, if available). Completely dry the feet and put on clean, non-skid socks and footwear if the client gets out of the bed.

- Clean up supplies, make the bed, and document the bath.

Showering

Many clients may prefer to shower rather than bathe in a tub. As with bathing, the water temperature should not exceed 110° F.

Before the shower begins, collect all necessary supplies including extra towels and washcloths. Wash your hands thoroughly, put on gloves, greet the client, verify his/her identity, let him/her know what you are going to be doing, and give him/her privacy. If there is any sign that the client does not want to shower at that time, respect his/her wishes and report it to the nurse.

Clients may need assistance getting in and/or out of the shower. A shower chair should be used if the client is unsteady or physically disabled in some way that affects his/her ability to safely stand. Ensure that the floor stays dry to avoid slipping and/or falling. Non-skid bath or shower mats are also highly important to prevent accidents.

Perineal Care

Perineal care is the care and cleaning of a client's genital and rectal areas. This cleaning is essential to ensure the prevention of infections, odors, and any irritation in those areas. Perineal care should be performed on a daily basis and more often when the client is incontinent. All incontinent clients must be washed and dried after each episode of incontinence. Patients should never be left wet or soiled because of incontinence.

It is also important to note that perineal care is completed on clients with and without a urinary catheter in place. Those with a urinary catheter require some extra steps.

For male clients without a urinary catheter:

- Fill a basin with water, no greater than 110° F.

- Position the patient on his back.

- Place a protective cover over the bed linen.

- Wash the groin from front to back, starting at the groin area and moving to the inside of the thighs.

- Rinse the washcloth or use a new one.

- Pull back the foreskin if the patient is not circumcised.

- Wash and rinse the tip of the penis downward while using gentle, circular motions and then the scrotum.

- Rinse the washcloth.

- Turn the patient on his side.

- Wash, rinse, and dry the rectal area.

For female patients without a urinary catheter:

- Fill the bath basin with clean water at 110° F.

- Position the patient on her back.

- Place a protective cover over the bed linen.

- Separate the outer labia and wash, rinse, and dry the urethral area with the inner labia. Use short, downward strokes alternating from side to side and proceeding until the exposed area around the urethra is done.

- Rinse the washcloth or use a new one.

- Wash the groin on the outside of the labia from front to back, starting outside the labia and moving to the inside of the thighs.

- Rinse the washcloth.

- Turn the patient on her side.

- Wash, rinse, and dry the rectal area.

Perineal care for male and female patients with a urinary catheter includes the above steps followed by these additional steps:

- With a clean washcloth and soap, wash the catheter with short strokes, starting at the urinary opening to about four inches away from the body.

- Using a new washcloth, rinse the catheter with short strokes, starting at the urinary opening to about four inches away from the body.

Shaving

Male clients often want to be shaven daily or every other day, whereas female clients may want to shave, or be shaven, every other day or weekly. Younger female clients typically prefer more frequent shaving of their legs and under arms than do older female clients. As with all other personal care needs, the nursing assistant and other members of the healthcare team should listen and accommodate the client's wants and needs. Additionally, always check with the nurse before shaving a client to ensure he/she is able to shave or be shaven by a nursing assistant. Some clients may have a disease, illness, or disorder or may be taking a medicine such as a blood thinner that can lead to poor clotting and bleeding.

Collect all necessary items you will need such as razors, shaving cream, basin of warm water, towels, and any other items the client may want. Wash your hands thoroughly and put on gloves. Greet the client, verify his/her identity, and let him/her know what you are going to be doing.

If the client is able to shave, but just needs some help, help him/her as needed. If the client is unable to shave at all, follow these steps:

- Raise the head of the bed if the person is allowed to be in a sitting position.

- Place a towel or protective barrier under the area to be shaved.

- If using an electric razor, follow the instructions. If using a regular razor, put warm water on the beard or hair to soften it.

- Shake the can of shaving cream.

- Place the shaving cream in your hand.

- Lather up the hair or beard with the shaving cream.

- Hold the skin so it is firm and tight.

- Gently shave a small area in the direction of the hair growth. For example, if shaving the side of the face, start at the side burn and shave downward. Shave upward when shaving the neck.

- Rinse the razor and repeat the previous step until the entire facial area is done.

- Wash and dry the area that has been shaved.

- Apply lotion or after-shave lotion if the patient desires.

- Clean all equipment and supplies.

- If any area was accidentally nicked, apply pressure to bleeding areas. Report and document all areas of bleeding.

The same steps are used when shaving a female client's legs and armpits. Shave small areas in the direction of the hair growth.

Oral Hygiene

Oral hygiene is yet another area that can be difficult for clients to manage. They may need help brushing and flossing their teeth; applying toothpaste to their toothbrush; and brushing their teeth, gums, and tongue without missing any areas including the inside and outside of the teeth. Good oral care is necessary to maintain health.

Dental Caries (Cavities)

There are many different types of bacteria in the mouth. When starches and sugars from different types of food and beverages mix with these bacteria, plaque forms on the teeth. Plaque's acid levels attack tooth enamel, which leads to dental caries, or cavities.

Some conditions that can lead to cavities include:
- A large amount of cavity-causing bacteria in the saliva
- A large amount of sugary and/or acidic foods and drinks consumed by the client
  - Sugar + plaque = cavities
  - Acid + plaque = cavities
- Poor oral hygiene habits such as not brushing and flossing
- Low fluoride exposure in drinking water and oral hygiene products such as toothpaste and mouthwashes
- Some medical conditions and medications that cause "dry mouth" (saliva is needed to rinse bacteria off teeth)

Signs and Symptoms

Some of the signs and symptoms of dental caries are pain and tooth sensitivity to sweets and/or cold foods and drinks.

Cavities can be detected:
- Visually - Cavities commonly appear as a brown or black spot, or it can start as a white spot.
- Manually - Cavities feel soft and sticky when a dentist probes them.
- X-rays and new technological advances, such as fluorescent lights or lasers, can also detect cavities and tooth areas that have lost minerals (demineralization).

When the cavities are small and have just small areas of demineralized enamel, the tooth can be filled or a special fluoride toothpaste or mouth rinse can be used. These dentist-ordered toothpastes and rinses can "remineralize" and harden the demineralized tooth.

When a cavity is medium to severe, it is treated by drilling away the soft decay and filling the tooth. Highly severe cavities are treated with a root canal to save the tooth. The infected nerve is removed with a root canal. The last alternative is extraction in which the entire tooth, including the infected inside area, is removed.

The nursing assistant and other healthcare workers should inform clients about ways to prevent cavities and other oral problems. Some topics that should be covered include:

- Diet:
  Clients should be instructed to limit the amount of sugary and/or acidic foods and drinks they consume.

- Oral Hygiene:
  Clients should be instructed to brush and floss their teeth at least twice a day, but more often whenever possible.

- Dry Mouth Correction:
  There are over-the-counter products and dentist-ordered products, such as Biotene and Therabreath, that can help eliminate dry mouth.

- Regular Dental Care:
  Clients should be instructed to get regular dental care, preferably twice a year, so their teeth can be professionally cleaned and cavities can be detected at the earliest stage by the dentist.

Gingivitis

If plaque is not removed from the client's teeth, it will harden under the gum line. This hardened plaque (called tartar or calculus) irritates, inflames, and damages the gingiva of the gums. It can also lead to swelling and bleeding of the gums. Tartar can be removed only with a professional dental cleaning.

The signs and symptoms of gingivitis include tender and/or bleeding gums; loose teeth; reddened, rather than pink, gums; pus between the gums and teeth; gums that recede and shrink; and bad breath.

Dentists diagnose gingivitis with measurements of the gums and x-rays. Dentists perform deep dental cleaning of the teeth to remove the plaque and tartar. Polishing is done after the cleaning to prevent further bacteria from sticking to the teeth. At times, an antibiotic treatment to heal the gums is also used. Severe cases may require gum surgery to treat the disease.

Left untreated, gingivitis can lead to a more serious infection known as advanced gum disease or periodontitis. This disorder destroys the soft tissue and bone that support the teeth; in time, this causes the gums to pull away from the teeth. This can then lead to the client's teeth becoming loose and falling out. Diabetics tend to suffer from a more severe type of periodontitis because diabetes causes the client to have a lower ability to resist infections; they are slow healers as well.

Toothbrushes

Toothbrushes can be soft, medium, or hard-bristled. A hard, or firm, toothbrush is sometimes used for serious dental needs, but it has disadvantages. The hard bristles may remove the protective enamel of the teeth and irritate the gums, particularly during vigorous brushing. Medium toothbrushes may be appropriate, at times, for people with a healthy mouth and teeth, but medium-bristled brushes also have disadvantages. A soft toothbrush is the best choice of all.

A soft toothbrush gently cleans and rids the teeth of soft plaque. It is also good for sensitive teeth, enamel loss, braces, and other conditions of the mouth. Hard and medium brushes lead to tooth sensitivity; since plaque is soft, a soft toothbrush is all that is needed to brush away all the soft plaque. Once the plaque turns hard and into tartar, it can't be brushed away with anything, not even with a medium or hard-bristled brush. So, again, a soft-bristled brush is recommended. A professional dental cleaning is the only way to rid the mouth of tartar.

In addition to the hard to soft categories of toothbrushes, there are other choices from which the client can choose:

- Manual toothbrushes

- Sonic toothbrushes are the most expensive of all toothbrushes on the market today, but they are good. The bristles move at a very fast rate of speed with a good vibrating motion so that plaque and staining are easily removed. Some come with an ultraviolet (UV) sanitizer and a timer so the client will know when he/she has completed the minimum two-minute tooth brushing session.

- Electric toothbrushes are quite like sonic toothbrushes, but they cost less and have fewer features. The motions of the bristles are consistent with the proper tooth brushing procedure.

- Foam toothbrushes are individually wrapped toothbrushes made of foam that have toothpaste on them. These foam brushes are good for travel and for people who are ill and cannot tolerate water and/or more complete mouth care.

Regardless of the client's choice, the client should always use an ADA-approved brand name toothbrush.

Toothbrushes make a very good hiding place for germs, and germs like wet surfaces. The client should be advised to always rinse the toothbrush after use and allow it to air dry in a clean environment. Toothbrushes should be discarded after a month of use.

Toothpastes

Some toothpastes have fluoride; others do not. Some have flavors; others do not. Some contain things like baking soda; others do not. Some are gels, and others are a paste or powder. Other than choosing fluoride toothpaste, the client should be instructed to purchase only toothpastes with an ADA approval on the packaging.

Some of the different kinds of toothpaste include:

- Tartar Control Toothpastes:
  These toothpastes do NOT remove tartar under the gums, but they can control it. Currently, only regular dental cleanings will remove tartar under the gums.

- Baking Soda Toothpastes:
  Although these products are probably not any more effective than others, many people like the squeaky clean feel after using them. However, clients should be aware that some baking soda toothpastes also contain peroxide, which can lead to gum damage and irritation.

- Smokers' Toothpastes:
  These products remove some of the tar and nicotine stains caused by cigarette smoking, but they are also abrasive. They can cause the gums to recede and can also remove some enamel. Smoking cessation is a much better alternative.

- Sensitive Teeth Toothpastes:
  These toothpastes are less abrasive than other products. They are helpful to those with a hot or cold tooth sensitivity, which can occur with dental caries, gum disease, and/or a tooth root exposure.

- Tooth-Whitening Toothpastes:
  These products have some limited effect on tooth whitening; however, they can also damage teeth.

Proper Tooth Brushing

At a minimum, all clients should be instructed to brush with fluoride toothpaste for at least two minutes at least three times a day.

The proper brushing technique is to hold the toothbrush at a 45° angle toward the gum line. The goal is to remove cavity and gum disease-causing plaque that may be hiding below the gums and on the teeth. All tooth surfaces, including the front and biting, and tongue surfaces are brushed. The insides of the cheeks and the entire tongue are also brushed.

Flossing

Flossing between teeth and under the gum line at least once a day with dental floss or an electronic cleaner will remove plaque that tooth brushing could not reach.

Some find the process of holding and manipulating the floss difficult and cumbersome. Pre-loaded floss handles sold by the bag are much easier to use and are just as effective as using traditional floss. Instead of wrapping the floss around the fingers, you simply hold the handle against the tooth to form a "C" around the tooth and then gently move the floss up and down in a vertical motion.

Clients lacking the fine motor skills to floss can benefit from a Waterpik® or an air flosser. They are just as good as using regular floss and are a lot easier.

Flossing must be a regular part of daily oral hygiene. The choices of dental floss and dental flossers are numerous. Any ADA-approved floss or device will do the job well, provided it is used properly and at least once a day.

Mouth Washing

The mouth is moist, warm, and dark—an excellent place for germs and bacteria to live, grow, multiply, and hide. They find tiny, comfortable hiding places between the teeth, along and under the gum line, on the insides of the cheeks, and on the tongue. All of these bacteria lead to plaque.

Germs and bacteria are loosened after tooth brushing and flossing, so the mouth should be vigorously rinsed to expel these germs. The physical force of moving a fluid, like water or mouthwash, forces these germs to loosen, and, with the addition of an antiseptic mouthwash, they can no longer grow and multiply.

Mouth washing should be done after each tooth brushing and flossing session and more often whenever possible.

Types of Mouthwashes

Some mouthwashes have alcohol; others do not. Some have fluoride; others do not. Some have tooth-whitening agents; others do not. Some contain an antiseptic; others do not. Some claim to treat the gums and avoid cavities; others do not make these same claims.

Many people select an alcohol-free mouthwash like Listerine Zero® because they dislike the taste of alcohol and/or are in a recovery program (like Alcoholics Anonymous) and cannot have any alcohol at all. The same is true for children, pregnant women, and nursing mothers. These populations should use only an alcohol-free mouthwash. However, since alcohol dries out tissues, including tissues in the mouth, plaque will more easily stick to teeth if an alcohol-containing mouthwash is used.

The next choice for clients is to determine whether or not to choose a mouthwash that contains fluoride. ACT® is an example of a mouthwash that contains fluoride. Fluoride fights cavities because it remineralizes the teeth.

Mouthwash is NOT a substitute for tooth brushing and flossing. It is an additional part of oral care.

Here are the steps for correctly using mouthwash:
- Dilute the mouthwash if the label states to do so.
- Designate an amount of the mouthwash that will fill about half of the mouth.
- Swish the mouthwash around the entire mouth so all surfaces are rinsed.
- Swish VIGOROUSLY for at least 30 seconds and up to one minute or more.

Denture Care

Some difficulties a client may experience with the care of dentures include cleaning them, inserting them, removing them, and applying the necessary adhesive to hold them in place properly.

Denture care is done before mouth care. If the client needs some or complete help with the care of his/her dentures, help them as needed. Follow these steps for denture care:

- With washed and gloved hands, remove or have the client remove his/her own dentures. If you are removing them, it is best to hold the upper denture and gently pull down and out of the mouth. To remove the lower denture, hold them and gently pull up and out of the mouth.

- Place the dentures in an emesis basin or denture cup.

- Line the sink with a paper towel or water to help avoid any denture breakage should you accidentally drop them.

- Run cool or room-temperature water. Do not use hot water; hot water can damage dentures.

- Rinse the dentures.

- Using a toothbrush and toothpaste, gently brush the dentures while holding them safely and firmly in your hand.

- Rinse the dentures under the running water.

- Place the dentures in a denture cup or emesis basin with cool water, mouthwash, or a denture-cleaning tablet until they are put back in the person's mouth after mouth care.

Dentures removed at nighttime must be cleaned and stored in a denture cup filled with water and a denture-cleaning tablet, which is used for disinfection. Label the denture cup with the client's full name and room number and store it in a safe place, such as a drawer or cabinet, so that the cup is not knocked over or misplaced. Dentures are often lost in healthcare facilities and are costly to replace, so nursing assistants must exercise care and caution when caring for dentures.

If you notice bad breath; abnormally tender or painful areas; chipped or broken teeth or dentures; coating of the tongue or cheeks; sores; or redness or bleeding in the mouth or on the gums, cheeks or lips, report it to the nurse and document it.

Foot Care

All clients have their feet washed as part of the bathing/showering process, but there is extra foot care that should also be provided. This form of care proves to be relaxing for the client and helps keep his/her feet soft and clean. When providing special foot care, follow these steps:

- Sit the client in a chair if possible. If he/she is on bed rest, foot care can be done by flexing the client's leg before completing this special care.

- Fill a wash basin with water that is about 110° F.

- Put a towel under the basin.

- Soak one of the client's feet in the basin for about 10 minutes.

- On the dry foot, gently push the cuticles back with a nail care stick.

- Clean under the nails with a nail care stick.

- If the toenails are to be cut, follow the steps in the Nail Care section of the "Dressing and Grooming" part of this chapter.

Cleaning and drying all parts of the foot, including between the toes, is important. If any abnormalities such as corns or bunions, bleeding, broken or chipped nails, or blue or pale nail beds are noticed, they should be promptly reported and documented.

DRESSING AND GROOMING

Dressing

Dressing is often very challenging for patients. Some clients have difficulties putting on and taking off clothing. They may lack the fine motor skills that are needed for fastening buttons, tying laces, and maneuvering zippers and other types of fasteners. Although there are a number of assistive devices that can help clients to dress independently, many clients do not have them when they are in a hospital for a short stay. In long-term care facilities, devices to facilitate a patient's independent dressing are often provided by the occupational therapist. For example, the client may have a long handled shoe horn so they can put their shoes on.

Hair Care

Patients can also experience difficulties with washing, conditioning, brushing and/or combing one's hair because they have problems with grasping, holding and manipulating a comb, brush, or styling device. It also takes considerable strength and skill to remove product tops by pulling, popping, or unscrewing them off and then getting the product out of the container with squeezing, pushing a button, scooping etc.

Hair can be washed in the shower, bathtub or in the bed using a special bed tray or a dry shampoo which is specially formulated to not require water.

Gather all necessary supplies, such as towels, shampoo, conditioner, and a wide-tooth comb, and then wash and dry your hands and apply protective gloves.

When shampooing a client's hair in the bed using a bed shampoo tray, the steps are:

- Cover the pillow with a towel or protective cover to keep it dry

- Put a towel under the person's neck and arms after untying the gown or loosening the bed clothing

- Put the bed shampoo pan under the person's head

- Place a washcloth over the person's eyes so the shampoo does not burn them. "Tearless" baby shampoo is very good to use when the patient has it.

- Check the temperature of the water to make sure it is about 110 degrees

- Pour a small amount of water on the hair using a water pitcher while keeping as much water as possible off the face

- Put a small amount of shampoo on the head

- Gently massage the hair and scalp with your fingertips. Do not use the fingernails. Fingernails can scratch the scalp.

- Rinse the head using water. Start at the top of the head and let the water work its way down to the bottom of the head.

- Repeat the rinsing and shampooing if needed

- Raise the person to a sitting position

- Dry the face

- Dry the head using a hair blower

- Change the gown or bed clothes if needed

- Clean up the area and place the person in a comfortable position with the bed in the lowest position

All clients should have their hair brushed/combed more than once a day in order to avoid matting or tangling. In the past many nursing assistants routinely cut patients' hair and braided it to avoid matting and tangling, however, this is not acceptable practice. Hair is cut and styled according to the client's wishes only.

When assisting a client with hair combing/brushing, there are certain steps that should be followed.

- Cover the pillow with a towel if the person is in bed.

- Gently comb or brush one section at a time. Do not pull on the hair. If the hair is tangled, comb the ends first and then work your way up to the scalp.

- Remove the towel and let the person see how they look using a mirror.

- Clean the brush or comb. Do not share combs or brushes among your clients.

If you observe bugs in the client's hair or on their body, scalp dryness, such as flaking or dandruff, sores, redness or bleeding, it must be reported and documented.

Nail Care

Client nail care is another important area of hygiene. The client's nails should to be checked daily for cleanliness and for any irregularities. The client's nails should be clean, trimmed short, and smooth without jagged surfaces.

Nail care is best performed when the client is sitting up in a chair but it can also be done when the patient is lying in bed. Toenails should never be cut on any clients who have diabetes, or problems with their circulation to their feet. You should always ask before performing toenail cutting because some facilities do not allow nursing assistants to cut client's toenails.

Before nail care is performed, you need to gather all necessary supplies, such as nail files, clippers, cuticle tools, and orange wood sticks to clean under the nails. The procedure is below.

- Fill a wash basin with water at about 110 degrees

- Put a towel under the basin

- Place the person's hand in the basin to soak them for about 10 minutes

- Gently push the cuticles back with a nail care stick while soaking the other hand or foot

- Clean under the nails with a nail care stick

- Trim the nails using a clipper

- File the edges with a nail file so that they are smooth

- Repeat the procedure for the other hand or foot

- Dry the hands or feet

- Apply lotion to the hands and feet avoiding the areas between the toes.

NUTRITION AND HYDRATION

According to the United States Department of Agriculture's "My Plate", the food groups are:
- Grains
- Vegetables
- Fruits
- Dairy
- Proteins

Grains can be whole or refined. Vegetables can be classified as dark green and red/orange and this food group also includes string beans, peas, starchy vegetables and other vegetables like artichokes, cabbage, lettuce, and peppers. The fruit group consists of a vast variety including bananas, pineapple, apples and grapes. Dairy products include milk, yogurt, all varieties of cheeses including soft cheeses like cottage cheese and hard cheeses like cheddar. The protein food group includes soy, nuts, seeds, beans, peas and other more commonly recognized sources of protein like meat, seafood or fish, eggs and poultry.

Some of the factors that impact on a client's nutritional status are:
- Culture
- Religion
- Appetite
- Finances
- Personal choices
- Bodily reactions to foods like aversions and food allergies
- Illnesses
- Medications
- Impaired Cognitive Functioning
- Chewing Problems
- Swallowing Problems
- Age
- Gender

For example, the age and development status of the client affects their nutritional needs. Adolescents require more calories than elderly people, because of their rapid stage of growth and development. Gender also affects nutritional preferences. For example, many women generally prefer to eat light soups or salads, whereas men usually prefer meat and potatoes.

Different ethnicities, cultures, as well as individuals within a culture can have different preferences regarding food. There may also be variances in terms of the amount of food consumed as well.

Furthermore, food and dietary preferences are also influenced by a client's belief about foods, such as eating a specific cereal because of a commercial or advertisement that offers better health. There are often religious beliefs that influence a client's diet as well. For example, Islam followers do not eat pork and some protestant religions forbid consuming alcohol, coffee, tea and meat.

Nutrition is also impacted by lifestyles. For example, those who work outside of the home may choose to eat fast foods, which are mostly unhealthy, because they do have the time or desire to cook when they come home from work.

Economic issues also impact a client's nutrition status. For example, some are unable to afford fresh fruits or vegetable. There are also clients who live without a stove and/or refrigerator, thus leaving the diabetic client with no choices other than eating out, which most often means that the client will eat less expensive fast foods rather than more expensive, but healthier, freshly prepared restaurant meals.

Health conditions, such as swallowing disorders affect a client's nutritional status. Other health disorders that can affect a client's nutritional status include nausea, vomiting, diarrhea, diabetes, hypertension, and a number of others. The assessment process includes assessing all of these factors.

Psychological disorders that can affect a client's nutritional status include anorexia and bulimia, which are most common in adolescent females. Depression, loneliness and stress also affect a client's nutritional status.

Many clients with physical diseases and disorders need a special diet. Some of the most commonly used special diets are:
- Clear Liquids
- Full Liquids
- Mechanical Soft Diet
- Fiber/Residue Restricted Diet
- High Fiber Diet
- Bland Diet
- High Calorie Diet
- Calorie Controlled Diet
- High Iron Diet

- Low-Cholesterol/Fat Controlled Diet
- High Protein Diet
- Sodium Controlled Diet
- Diabetes Diet
- Dysphagia Diet

Enteral and Parenteral Nutrition

Enteral nutrition delivers nourishment and nutrients directly into the gastrointestinal tract with a tube feeding like a nasogastric tube feeding or a gastrostomy tube feeding. Some at the end of life choose to have enteral or parenteral nutrition and others elect to forgo this form of nutrition. These artificial forms of nutrition, when used, are most often given to clients with severe gastrointestinal disorders such as cancer and malabsorption.

The types of enteral nutrition are:
- Nasogastric Tube (NG Tube)
- Gastrostomy Tube

Some of the complications of enteral nutrition include diarrhea and aspiration. The nursing assistant should monitor and report client responses to enteral nutrition and prevent aspiration by positioning the client and observing the client for comfort and delayed gastric emptying during the process of feeding.

Unlike enteral nutrition, parenteral nutrition is delivered intravenously. This method is preferred when the client needs, and chooses to, have nutritional support for more than one week. Although this form of nutrition can be delivered through a peripheral vein, it is most often delivered with a central venous catheter and a port. . Scrupulous sterile dressing changes must be done by the nurse in order to prevent infection which is a commonly occurring complication of parenteral nutrition.

Helping Clients to Eat and Drink

Clients often need help with eating and drinking. They may have problems such as cutting their food and getting food onto a fork or spoon. They may also have trouble with chewing and swallowing.

As a nursing assistant, you play an important role in helping a client to meet their nutrition and hydration needs. Clients can suffer from poor nutrition and/or dehydration if they are not receiving the necessary vitamins, minerals, nutrients and proteins from consumed food and/or fluids, especially when they are ill or have an infection.

Water and fluids are a necessity in all people. The body is made up of mostly water. Fluids control the temperature of the body, they keep the body's cells alive and they keep the blood flowing. Fluids can be found in foods and fluids like tea, coffee, juice and plain water.

If a client does not get enough fluid in their body they can become dehydrated. The signs and symptoms of dehydration are:

- Eyes that appear sunken
- Dry skin
- Skin that is loose with poor skin turgor
- Dry mouth and dry tongue
- Confusion
- Fever
- Nausea
- Vomiting
- Lack of interest
- Weakness
- Lack of appetite
- Constipation
- Low blood pressure
- Weak and fast pulse rate
- Dark urine
- Less than normal urinary output
- Dizziness when going from a lying to standing position
- Weight loss

The steps for feeding a client are:

- Prepare the patient or resident for his/her meal. Wash or ask the patient to wash his/her hands and face. Ask the patient if he/she would like to use the bathroom, commode, urinal, or bedpan before eating.

- Wash your hands before and after feeding each patient or resident. Some assisted living and nursing homes have sinks in the dining areas. Others may use a waterless hand washing product for frequent hand washing.

- Keep the dining room or patient room bright, cheerful, clean, and free from bad odors.

- Place the patient or resident in a comfortable and safe position. Chairs in the dining room should be comfortable. People in wheelchairs should be placed at the table so they can reach their food and drink. If the patient is eating in his/her bed, the head of the bed should be up at least 30° so the patient can safely swallow food and fluids. Over-the-bed tables must be clean and put in place so the patient can see and reach his/her meal.

- Give the patient his/her meal and check to make sure he/she is getting the correct meal. Some clients have special diets.

- Check the food temperatures. Cold foods should be cold, and hot foods should be warm, but not hot enough to cause a burn.

- Place the meal so the patient can reach it, if he/she can safely do so.

- Help the patient with his/her meal as much as needed.

- Feed patients and residents that must be fed. Feed them slowly. Tell them what they are eating. Talk with them and give them time between bites so they can enjoy their food. If a patient cannot use one side of his/her face or mouth, put the food and drinking straw on the other side of his/her mouth. Tell patients to swallow and provide other cues, as needed.

- Alternate foods if the client is unable to tell you which food he/she would like to eat. For example, feed the patient some meat, then some vegetables, then some milk, and then, perhaps, some bread or potatoes. Feed them at the speed in which they want to eat. Use a different straw for each fluid. Do NOT force a patient to eat something he/she does not want to eat. Encourage patients and residents to eat, but NEVER force anyone if he/she does not want to eat.

- Check, record, and report how much and what the patient has eaten. Write down the person's name and how much meat, peas, potatoes, and milk (or other fluid) he/she has eaten. If the patient has not eaten well, immediately report it to the nurse in charge.

- Return the patient to his/her room and clean him/her up if needed. Clean crumbs and food off the bed if the patient has eaten his/her meal in the bed.

- Keep the patient or resident in a sitting position for at least 30 minutes after the meal, so he/she does not choke.

Some patients, particularly older people, are not able to cut their meat; use a fork, knife and spoon; and/or open their milk container and place a straw in it. Some people need only a small amount of help to open their milk or cut their meat, for example. Others, however, need much more help in order to consume a good diet. Most often, nursing assistants provide this needed help.

People with blindness or poor vision need help eating too. They may require help cutting their food, opening their drinks, and some other special help. Nursing assistants should tell these patients and residents where the food is on their plate. The best way to do this is by using the clock method. For example, patients could be told that the potatoes are at 9 o'clock, the hamburger is at 3 o'clock, and the carrots are at 6 o'clock.

Some patients and residents may also have a swallowing problem. They can choke on foods and can't drink liquids such as water, juice, tea, or coffee safely. Nurses often ask nursing assistants to give these patients water and fluids made as thick as honey in order to prevent choking.

Others are completely dependent on others to feed them; they can't feed themselves at all. Patients should be allowed and encouraged to be as independent as possible. Independence makes a person feel good, and it maintains his/her sense of dignity and self-worth.

Sources of Intake and Output

Intake consists of solids (foods) and fluids. Fluid intake includes:
- Water
- Milk
- Coffee and tea
- Soups
- Ices
- Jello

Fluid output includes:
- Vomitus
- Diarrhea
- Urine
- Wound drainage
- Other losses such as perspiration

Measuring Intake and Output

Fluid Intake and Output Measurements
- 1 ounce = 30 ml
- 1 pint = 500 ml
- 1 quart = 1,000 ml

Solid Output Measurements
- Number of BMs per day
- Diaper counts for infants and neonates

ELIMINATION

Some clients may have problems associated with elimination including constipation, hemorrhoids, diarrhea, and managing bowel and/or bladder incontinence. Many clients with (and without) these problems may also need assistance with toileting. For example, they may require help getting to the bathroom or commode, and they may need assistance with wiping.

Urinary Elimination

Normal urine is clear, yellow, odorless, and without any particles or blood. People normally void about 1,500 cc of urine per day; however, the volume and characteristics of urine produced and the manner in which it is expelled can be affected by a variety of factors such as:

- Age:
  Older adults can experience problems with urinary elimination due to the aging process. Older men can have enlarged prostate glands, which can lead to urinary incontinence and urinary retention due to the inability to empty the entire bladder. Older women, particularly after experiencing menopause, can experience urgency and stress incontinence as a result of decreased perineal tone and weakened support of the bladder, vagina, and supporting tissues.

- Psychosocial Factors:
  The micturition, or voiding, reflex is stimulated with normal positioning, privacy, and enough time. When clients are without these factors, they may be unable to physically relax enough to void. Other clients may feel anxious or rushed and therefore, cannot void either.

- Fluid and Food Intake:
  Foods high in sodium can cause a client to retain water and therefore, prevent them from voiding. In many cases, increasing fluid intake will increase fluid output.

- Medications:
  A number of medications can affect the body's normal urination process. For example, diuretics, or "water pills," increase urine formation and output. The color of the urine can also be altered by certain medications.

- Muscle Tone:
  Clients with poor bladder muscle tone often require a retention catheter. The muscle tone in the pelvic region can also affect a client's ability to store and empty urine.

- Pathologic Conditions:
  Urine formation and excretion can be affected by a variety of diseases and pathogens. The ability of the nephrons to produce urine can be affected by diseases of the kidney such as renal failure in which the kidneys stop producing urine. Blood flow to the kidneys and good kidney health can also be adversely affected by heart and circulatory disorders such as shock, heart failure, and hypertension. Processes that interfere with urine flow from the kidneys to the urethra can also affect urinary excretion. For example, hypertrophy of the prostate can impair urination and bladder emptying because it can obstruct the urethra.

Some urinary disorders are:

- Polyuria:
  Polyuria is an excessive amount of urine produced by the kidneys, which can occur among those with a history of diabetes mellitus, diabetes insipidus, and kidney

disease. Polyuria can lead to dehydration, excessive thirst, and weight loss as a result of excessive fluid loss.

- Oliguria:
Oliguria is a less than normal amount of urinary output. Oliguria can result from decreased fluid intake, excessive fluid loss, impaired blood flow to the kidneys, and renal failure.

- Anuria:
Anuria is a lack of the production of urine.

- Dysuria:
Dysuria is painful or difficult urination. It can result from a urinary tract infection or trauma.

- Urinary Incontinence:
Urinary incontinence is an involuntary leakage of urine and a loss of bladder control. This is more common in women, due to childbirth, which can cause trauma to the pelvic floor, a shorter urethra, and menopause. As a result, women often have stress incontinence, which is urinary leakage that occurs when a person coughs, sneezes, or laughs. Cognitive impairments, decreased mobility, urinary tract infections, cerebrovascular accidents, spinal cord injury, and other diseases and disorders can also lead to urinary incontinence.

Managing urinary incontinence includes bladder training, which is also referred to as continence training; pelvic muscle exercises; maintaining skin integrity; and using external urinary drainage devices and briefs. Whenever possible, indwelling urinary catheters should be avoided because they can lead to infections.

- Urinary Retention:
Urinary retention is a condition in which urine accumulates in the bladder and distends it. It often occurs when a client is unable to completely empty his/her bladder.

The first steps in treating urinary retention include maintaining adequate fluid intake, maintaining normal voiding habits, and giving the client needed assistance with toileting. If these actions aren't successful, the doctor may prescribe a cholinergic drug, which can help stimulate bladder contractions and allow more complete bladder emptying.

Bowel Elimination

Some of the factors that affect bowel elimination include level of development, diet, activity, psychological factors, defecation habits, medications, diagnostic procedures, anesthesia and surgery, pathologic conditions, and pain.

Common problems with fecal elimination include constipation, which is having fewer than three bowel movements a week; fecal impaction, which is a mass or collection of hardened feces within the folds of the rectum; diarrhea; bowel incontinence; and flatulence, which results from swallowed air, gas that diffuses between the bloodstream and the intestine, or bacteria acting on the chyme in the large intestine.

The following interventions can help clients to defecate on a regular basis:
- Positioning
- Exercising
- Nutrition and fluids (fiber and fluids are helpful)
- Timing
- Privacy

Enemas

The four types of enemas are:

- Cleansing Enema:
  Cleansing enemas are used to remove feces. The usual reasons for this type of enema are to eliminate the presence of feces during surgery or a diagnostic test such as a colonoscopy and to remove feces in a client with constipation or impaction.

- Carminative Enema:
  A carminative enema is used primarily to expel flatus. With this type of enema, the fluid in the rectum expels gas.

- Retention Enema:
  With a retention enema, an oil solution or medication is introduced into the rectum and sigmoid colon, and it remains there for one to three hours. This type of enema is used to soften the feces and to lubricate the rectum and anal canal, which allows for easier passage of feces.

- Return-Flow Enema:
  A return-flow enema, also known as a Harris flush, is also used to expel flatus. The fluid is inserted into the rectum and sigmoid colon in order to stimulate peristalsis.

Ostomies

A colostomy is an ostomy made in the colon that diverts fecal contents. Colostomies can be permanent or temporary. They are performed in order to relieve a bowel obstruction caused by a tumor, to help promote the healing of anastomoses, and to eliminate bowel contents when the distal colon and rectum are removed.

There are different types of colostomies, named according to the portion of the colon where they are formed. They are categorized as ascending colostomy, transverse colostomy, descending colostomy, or sigmoid colostomy. The location of the stoma depends on what type/location of colostomy is performed. For example, the stoma is usually located on the lower left quadrant of the abdomen with a sigmoid colostomy.

REST/SLEEP/COMFORT

Rest, sleep, and comfort are essential for all clients. Several factors affect both quantity and quality of sleep. Quantity of sleep refers to the total time a person sleeps; quality of sleep refers to how energetic and refreshed the person feels when he/she awakens.

Some of these factors include:

- Illness:
  When a person suffers from an illness, his/her sleep is often affected during the time when sleep and rest are essential for health and healing. Sometimes, the patient may find it difficult to attain and retain comfort because he/she may be experiencing pain or physical distress from illness.

- Environment:
  A change in one's environment can negatively affect the amount and quality of sleep. For example, hospital environments are often noisy, so it is important for healthcare workers to take extra care in keeping hallways and units quiet so patients can relax, fall asleep, and stay asleep longer. Room temperature and the level of lighting can also impair sleep. Nurses and nursing assistants should ensure that the client environment is conducive to sleep and rest.

- Lifestyle:
  Exercise is important for sleep, but if a person exercises too late in the day, it can cause problems with his/her sleeping. In order to fall asleep, relaxation must be achieved; therefore, any exercise, work, or even eating close to bedtime can be problematic. Most patients should be able to exercise in some form. Walking, moving about in a wheelchair, and even arm and leg exercises in bed can improve sleep for many clients.

- Emotional Stress:
  The National Sleep Foundation states that stress is the leading cause of sleep problems. Stress makes it more difficult to relax; therefore, stress can lead to problems involving both sleep induction and sleep maintenance. Nurses and nursing assistants can relieve client stress by promoting stress management techniques and other nursing measures such as back rubs and soft music.

- Stimulants and Alcohol:
  When consumed in the late afternoon or evening, caffeine can interfere with a person's sleep.

- Diet:
  A person usually experiences a reduction in total sleep time as a result of weight gain, whereas a person who has lost weight tends to have an increase in total sleep time and a decrease in the number of times he/she awakens during the night.

- Smoking:
  In most cases, smokers have more problems sleeping than those who do not smoke. Nicotine acts as a stimulant, thus causing difficulties in falling asleep.

- Medications:
  A number of medication types can affect quantity and quality of sleep.

Common sleep disorders include:

- Insomnia:
  Insomnia is the most common sleep disorder in the U.S. Insomnia is an inability to fall asleep (sleep induction) or to remain asleep (sleep maintenance). This disorder leaves the person feeling as though he/she has not gotten enough rest. Acute insomnia can last for one to a few days, and it often results from excessive stress or worrying. Chronic insomnia is when this condition lasts over a month. People with any form of insomnia may experience irritability, concentration problems, daytime sleepiness, and feelings of inadequate rest.

- Hypersomnia:
  Hypersomnia is a condition in which a person is unable to stay awake during the daytime despite getting enough restful sleep at night. It is usually caused by a medical condition such as hypothyroidism or diabetic acidosis. In most cases, hypersomnia is unrelated to any psychological problems or disorders.

- Sleep Apnea:
  Sleep apnea consists of pauses in a person's breathing that occur frequently throughout the night. These periods of apnea can occur five or more times per night, and the duration can last for ten seconds or longer every hour.

  The symptoms of sleep apnea include excessive daytime sleepiness, snoring, several sudden awakenings throughout the night, irritability, morning headaches, memory and cognitive problems, and difficulties falling asleep.

  The treatment for sleep apnea depends on the cause. For example, if the apnea is related to enlarged tonsils, the tonsils can be removed. Other treatments include use of a CPAP device, laser removal of excessive tissue in the pharynx, and weight loss.

  Addressing sleep apnea is important. Left untreated, it can cause a sharp rise in blood pressure, which can lead to cardiac arrest, and other heart problems.

The promotion of sleep often depends on correcting the problem that causes sleep disruption. Addressing the cause and making changes can often be all that is necessary. Use of sleep medications should be used only as a last resort.

Setting a regular bedtime and wake time is important. Napping should be avoided by younger people with insomnia; for older adults, naps should be limited to a maximum of 15-30 minutes.

Getting a sufficient amount of daily exercise during the early part of the day is helpful.

The bed and bedroom should be relaxing and conducive to sleep. Ensuring the temperature and lighting encourage sleep and keeping a quiet atmosphere can contribute to this.

Chapter 2: Physical Care Skills—Basic Nursing Skills

INFECTION CONTROL

The Cycle of Infection

Infections can spread from person to person when germs:
- Are able to leave the body
- Have a means of transportation
- Can enter another body

Germs are everywhere: in the air; on and in our body; on our clothes; on and in food and liquids; in human waste; on table tops, bed sheets, and flowers; and everywhere else.

Nursing assistants can do many things to prevent the spread of germs. For example, nursing assistants must keep foods safe, keep patient rooms clean and without dust that carries germs through the air, and wash their hands to prevent the spread of infection.

Nursing assistants cannot prevent germs from leaving someone's body. Germs will leave a person's body when he/she coughs, sneezes, moves his/her bowels, and has a draining wound. Nursing assistants cannot control those things, but they can control the facial tissues used for sneezing and coughing. Tissues must be discarded in the correct manner.

Like tissues, hands are also vehicles for germs. Tissues, hands, and all other items that have, or may have, bodily fluids can move germs from one person to another. The spread of infection can be stopped when germs' transportation is removed.

The cycle of infection and transportation of infections can be eliminated when:
- Hands are washed properly before and after EVERY patient contact
- Hands are washed properly before and after EACH task
- All items that may, or may not, have germs are handled in the proper way
- Practices such as keeping dirty bed sheets away from our clothing are followed

EVERYONE must control infection!

Germs require darkness and moisture to live and multiply. When fed and given a dark and moist place to live, germs will grow and multiply out of control.

Nosocomial Infections

Nosocomial infections are infections that a patient did not have before being hospitalized, or cared for, but acquired after admission or after care was provided. Most nosocomial infections are spread from healthcare workers to patients via hand contact.

The most commonly occurring risk factors for nosocomial infections are prolonged illness and immunosuppression, which can result from an infection such as HIV, treatments such as chemotherapy, and some medications. Additionally, all equipment and non-sterile supplies can harbor and spread nosocomial infections. Some bacteria can even resist antibiotics. Nosocomial infections are quite costly, but they can, for the most part, be prevented.

The urinary tract, respiratory tract, wounds, and bloodstream are the most common sites for nosocomial infections. Some of the commonly occurring pathogens include:

- E. coli
- Candida albicans
- Staphylococcus aureus
- Pseudomonas aeruginosa
- Enterococcus

Hand washing is the single most effective way to prevent nosocomial infections in healthcare facilities. Protective precautions such as standard precautions and transmission-based precautions are also necessary to prevent the spread of these deadly infections. This prevention is extremely important because of the presence of so many resistant strains of pathogens such as methicillin-resistant staphylococcus aureas (MRSA), vancomycin-resistant enterococcus (VRE), and penicillin-resistant streptococcus pneumoniae.

Infections are serious and can even be extremely dangerous. Germs are all over, and infections can spread quickly in hospitals and other healthcare environments. Clients in a healthcare facility live closely together with other clients who are ill; therefore, they are more likely to get infections there than they would in their own home.

Some clients also have a weak immune system because they are elderly or an infant or as the result of AIDS/HIV or cancer treatment. These patients are at great risk for infection because their weak immune system cannot fight off infections like other healthy and unaffected immune systems can. For example, an elderly immune system will weaken over time; an infant has an undeveloped immune system; and AIDS/HIV, and other illnesses, weakens an immune system so infections can be very serious when contracted. Some infections can even lead to death.

Some areas of the hospital especially threatened by germs include:

- Kidney (or renal) areas, as these patients are more prone to infection
- Operating rooms, which must be sterile
- Labor and delivery
- Infant nursery
- ICU (intensive care units) and other special care areas

These areas often restrict the number of people in these areas so the number of germs can be controlled and reduced. For example, only operating room staff members are permitted in the operating room, and a small, limited number of people are permitted in a labor room when a baby is being born.

Intact, unbroken skin is the body's first line of defense against infections. All broken skin can lead to infection. For example, a person who has a pressure ulcer or an incision and stitches after surgery is at risk for infection because his/her skin is broken and not intact. All clients with an open wound must have a sterile dressing put on the area so that germs are unable to enter the body.

Drug Resistance

Germs can learn how to grow and change so they can resist antibiotics that used to be effective. This new growth pattern is called drug resistance and occurs because antibiotics have been abused and used too much. For example, many people needlessly take antibiotics for the flu or a cold. As stated previously, antibiotics do not cure viruses such as the flu or a cold, so this abuse of antibiotics leads to drug-resistant germs and pathogens.

As a result of this resistance, antibiotics are unable to work anymore and become useless. This is true, for example, with tuberculosis (TB) and staph infections. In addition to this problem, many antibiotic drugs are also found in common, everyday items such as water, food, and some soaps.

This resistance is dangerous not only for the client with the infection, but also for others. This is true because the affected client can spread germs to others who are then also unable to be cured since the germ is resistant to antibiotics.

This methicillin-resistant staphylococcus aureus (MRSA) germ is one of the most drug-resistant germs. MRSA quickly spreads from one person to another, and unfortunately, antibiotics are not always able to cure it because the germ has become resistant to the antibiotic methicillin.

MRSA can be transmitted unknowingly. It is more prevalent in hospitals and other healthcare facilities, but it can be contracted anywhere. For example, young children and people who play contact sports such as football and basketball and those who live in crowded places such as group homes, college dorms, and prisons are at risk for MRSA outside of healthcare facilities. In the hospital and other healthcare facilities, patients who are elderly, weak, have serious diseases and/or a poor immune system, and have lines or tubes in their body (intravenous lines and feeding tubes) are at risk for MRSA.

MRSA is a serious infection that can cause severe illness and sometimes, death. It starts with small red bumps on the skin and eventually turns in an abscess, which can or cannot spread to other areas in the body such as bones, heart, blood, and other parts.

Most people do not get sick from MRSA, but those who have a weakened immune system and are not strong enough to fight it off can get very sick from it. MRSA is often diagnosed when the patient has the signs of infection: redness, warmth, fever, swelling, soreness, and/or pus or another fluid coming from an open wound. This infection is often found when a skin or nasal sample is analyzed by a laboratory.

Currently, some antibiotics can still fight MRSA for some people; others can't.

Standard Precautions and Protective Precautions

- *Standard precautions* apply to all blood and bodily fluids and all clients, regardless of the person's diagnosis.

- *Contact precautions* prevent any direct and indirect contact transmissions, as can occur with diarrhea, wounds, and skin infections. Contact precautions are used when the client has an infection that can be transmitted through touch. It is necessary to wear a gown and gloves and use special soap when contact precautions are in place.

- *Airborne precautions* are used to prevent airborne transmission microbes such as tuberculosis (TB). Airborne precautions require the use of a special mask, called a HEPA mask, and a special negative pressure room.

- *Droplet precautions* are used to prevent the transmission of pathogens that are transmitted with a cough, sneeze, body fluid spray, etc. These clients are placed in a private room or a room with someone infected with the same microorganism. A mask, in addition to hand washing, is required when you enter the room of a patient who is on droplet precautions.

Special transmission precautions are used in addition to standard precautions when a client has an infection that is hard to control.

Standard precautions must be followed by all nursing assistants and other members of the healthcare team. Standard precautions require that all people, regardless of whether or not they have an infection, are treated the same by the nursing assistant and others. It is assumed that all people could be infected, so gloves and other personal protective equipment must be used when touching any bodily fluids. Some of these bodily fluids include urine; blood; feces; sputum; wound drainage; vomit; breast milk; and other fluids from the nose, lungs, or abdomen. For example, gloves must be worn when emptying a urinary drainage bag because urine may touch the hands; you should wear protective eye wear, gloves, and a gown when it is possible that bodily fluids may spray into the air. All of these bodily fluids could contain disease-causing germs, and you do not want these germs to enter your body or remain on your clothes or hands. When germs get on your clothes or hands, you will spread these germs to patients as you move from room to room.

According to the U.S. Centers for Disease Control and Prevention (CDC), infections are a very serious problem in healthcare. Infections are costly, overextend a patient's length of stay in the hospital, lower the person's quality of life, and cause pain and suffering to the patient and family members. Again, infection control and prevention must be a regular part of the nursing assistant's job.

Hand Washing

Hand washing is the MOST important thing that can be done in order to prevent the spread of infection. Dirt can be seen on our hands and nails, but germs are invisible to the naked eye. If your hands look clean, that doesn't mean they are germ-free. Hand washing is the number one way to prevent the spread of germs and infection. Also, keeping your finger nails trimmed and short helps to keep dirt and germs from hiding under them.

Your must wash your hands:
- As soon as you arrive at work
- Before you enter a patient's room
- Before you leave a patient' room
- Before you put on gloves and as soon as you remove them
- Before and after you touch anyone
- Before and after you perform any task
- Before and after you take a break
- Before you leave the restroom
- After you handle trash
- After you blow your nose, cough, or sneeze
- Before and after you eat or handle food
- When you leave work

The proper way to wash your hands is important, and it should take only about 20 seconds. Singing the "Happy Birthday" song twice takes about 20 seconds. For proper hand washing, follow these steps:

- Turn on the water.

- Wet your hands up to your wrists.

- While the water is running, apply a good amount of soap to your hands and wrists.
-
- Rub together your hands to get the soap full of suds.

- Hold down your hands, but do not touch the sink. Rub them for at least 15 seconds or so, making sure to include the front and back of your hands, in between your fingers, under your nails, and up to your wrists. If the soap starts to dry up, add just a small amount of water.

- Thoroughly rinse off your hands under the running water.

- Take a paper towel and dry off your hands.

- Turn off the faucet using the paper towel, NOT your hands.

- Throw away the paper towel.

If you forget or skip a step, start over again beginning with the first step. Keeping your hands clean and ensuring that the client is clean are two very important ways to protect against infection.

Personal Protective Equipment

All healthcare workers must use personal protective equipment to protect themselves and their clients. Gloves, gowns, masks, eye wear such as goggles, shoe covers, hair coverings, and HEPA masks (used when the patient has TB) are examples of personal protective equipment.

Gloves:
You MUST wear gloves every time you come into contact with bodily fluids or if there is a possibility for contact. For example, you must wear gloves when emptying a urine bag, urinal, or bed pan. You must remove these gloves when you are done with the task and dispose of them in the proper manner. Soiled gloves are considered biohazardous waste because they have been contaminated with bodily fluids, and they must be disposed of in a special red bag used for biohazardous waste.

You must also wash your hands after you remove the gloves. Gloves are NEVER used more than once; they are disposed of after each use. Also, gloves are discarded in the patient's room. NEVER walk around the halls with used gloves; this spreads infection.

Gowns:
You must wear a gown when doing something that may soil your clothes with bodily fluids. For example, put on a gown when bathing a client who has had an episode of diarrhea that has saturated the bed sheets and client's bed clothes. Gowns can be made of plastic or paper. Wear a plastic gown when the body secretion is wet. A plastic gown prevents wet bodily fluids from permeating the gown and soiling your clothes or uniform.

As soon as you are done with the task, remove the gown, discard it as biohazardous waste, and wash your hands.

Masks:
Simple surgical masks protect against fluids and droplets that can be splashed or sprayed into the mouth and nose. They also protect the client from the sneezes and coughs of healthcare workers. Masks are worn when the patient is infected with a respiratory disorder that can be spread through coughing and sneezing; they are also used in sterile environments such as the operating room. These masks protect against many airborne particles, but they are ineffective against TB.

High efficiency particulate absorption (HEPA) masks, also called respirators, are used in a variety of workplaces and industries including healthcare when a client has tuberculosis. Since regular surgical masks are ineffective against TB, healthcare facilities are required to fit staff for these special masks if they will be caring for TB patients.

Negative pressure rooms are also used for TB patients. Negative pressure pulls air into the TB patient's room from the hallway and prevents air from the patient's room from escaping into the hallway where other people could become infected with the TB.

Eye Protection & Face Shields:
Eye protection and face shields are used when a patient-care activity may involve a splash or spray of bodily fluids. These splashes and sprays most often occur in special care areas where activities such as suctioning are being done.

Like all other personal protective equipment, eye protection and face shields should be removed after use and discarded unless the equipment is intended for long-term use.

Biohazardous Waste Disposal

Used needles and other supplies and equipment are biohazardous when contaminated with blood or other bodily fluids. Used needles and other biohazardous wastes can transmit diseases, some of which can be life-threatening such as hepatitis and HIV/AIDS.

Biohazardous waste can be classified as either sharps (needles) or non-sharps (soiled dressings). Soiled dressings and other non-sharp wastes can be disposed of in the community and in healthcare settings. Red bags are used for the disposal of biohazardous waste in the healthcare setting. Sharps in the healthcare and community settings are disposed of in hard, red biohazardous waste containers.

Disposal of needles and other sharps in the home and community can be dangerous and is a public health risk. For example, public waste workers can encounter a needle or other sharp if it is discarded with the regular trash. Used needles can transmit diseases, and some can be life-threatening.

The U.S. Environmental Protection Agency collaborates with the Coalition for Safe Community Needle Disposal to offer solutions for the safe disposal of needles, syringes, and other sharps in all areas of the community including healthcare facilities. Some of these solutions include sharps collection sites and "mail return" sharps programs.

Other Infection Control Procedures

You must not sit on patient beds or chairs because you could spread infection to other patients. Soiled linen should not be placed against the body or work clothing or tossed on the floor; it should be discarded according to procedure. Clean linen should always be covered, not left exposed to the air.

The environment, patient furniture, and assistive devices must be kept clean and dust-free.

Blood-borne Pathogens

Some infections and diseases that are transmitted via blood and bodily fluids are:
- HIV
- Hepatitis type B
- Hepatitis type C

HIV/AIDS

The etiology of human immunodeficiency virus (HIV) is caused by the HIV-1 and HIV-2 retroviruses that deplete helper T-4 cells. This compromises cellular immunity.

These infections can range from primary asymptomatic infection to overt AIDS, which is often complicated with opportunistic infections that can lead to death. Opportunistic infections can affect the pulmonary system, nervous system, and musculoskeletal system. Some opportunistic infections include Kaposi's sarcoma, pneumocystis carinii pneumonia, candidiasis, cytomegalovirus, herpes simplex, and histoplasmosis.

Signs and symptoms of HIV/AIDS include fever, malaise, dyspnea, lethargy, skin rash, chills, night sweats, dry cough, oral lesions, diarrhea, weight loss, abdominal discomfort, headaches, stiff neck, confusion, swollen lymph glands, progressive edema, and seizures.

Highly active antiretroviral therapy (HAART) is used to treat HIV/AIDS. The goals of this treatment are to decrease the viral load, prevent secondary infections, and maintain the client in the best possible level of health. Compliance is critical to the success of this treatment because these medications must be taken for life, are expensive, and are associated with troublesome side effects.

Hepatitis Type B and Hepatitis Type C

Viral hepatitis is a major liver infection both in the U.S. and across the globe. Like HIV/AIDS, hepatitis is spread through blood and other bodily fluids.

Generally, all except necessary medications are avoided because the liver metabolizes medications. Chronic hepatitis C is treated with interferon; at times, vitamin K may be needed for prolonged prothrombin times.

SAFETY AND EMERGENCIES

Safety is a major priority in healthcare. Safety needs are the second priority after physical needs, according to Maslow's Hierarchy. According to Maslow, human needs (from highest to lowest priority) are:

- Physiological or Biological Needs:
  Physiological needs include hunger, thirst, sleep/rest, etc. Of all of these physiological needs, the need for the ABCs (airway, breathing, and cardiovascular function) is the greatest and highest priority.

- Safety and Psychological Needs:
  The need for safety, comfort, freedom from pain, and psychological comfort are included in this level.

- Love and Belonging:
  This level reflects a person's need for love and belonging. Humans want to be accepted by others and become, and remain, part of a group.

- Self-Esteem and Esteem by Others:
  Esteem needs reflect a person's need to achieve, be competent, gain approval and recognition from others (esteem), and have his/her own feelings of self-worth and self-esteem.

- Self-Actualization:
  Self-actualization reflects a client's need to reach his/her highest level of ability and potential. This level is not always achieved by an individual in his/her lifetime.

Preventing Medical Errors and Mistakes

Unfortunately, too many errors and mistakes occur in healthcare. These errors and mistakes are not necessarily intentional mistakes, but nonetheless, they do happen and too often.

Errors and mistakes can be classified as errors of omission or commission. Mistakes of omission are mistakes that occur because someone does not do what he/she is supposed to do. A nursing assistant who forgets to take a client's vital signs or to report rectal bleeding has committed an error of omission.

Errors of commission are mistakes that occur because someone does the wrong thing. A nursing assistant who takes in the wrong client for a procedure because he/she failed to check the patient's identification bracelet has committed an error of commission.

Mistakes and errors are an unfortunate problem and can occur anywhere healthcare is administered including hospitals, nursing homes, long-term care facilities, and even the client's home.

Some examples of high-risk areas for mistakes include:

- Broken and/or Faulty Medical Equipment:
  If any patient-care equipment is broken or does not seem to be working correctly, STOP using it immediately. The supervisor should be notified immediately if there is anything broken or not working correctly.

- Restraints:
  Restrained clients must be closely monitored to ensure they don't injure themselves or others. If asked to apply restraints, make sure you are competent and able to do so. Always report to the nurse if you are unable to, untrained to, or need help with anything you are asked to do. It is always better to be safe than sorry. If you have questions or have difficulty performing a task, always ask for assistance.

- Wandering and Elopement:
  Some clients are confused; therefore, they are at risk for harm or injury. These clients are at risk for wandering to places within the facility or even outside it, which is known as elopement. It is especially important to monitor these clients and to immediately respond to calls for help, bed alarms, and exit door alarms.

- Suicide:
  Clients at risk for suicide are to be on 24-hour watch. If asked to watch any of these clients, you must watch them at all times. There should never be a moment in which your eyes are not focused on the client.

In general, healthcare is at risk for errors. Many things can help prevent and stop these mistakes and errors, which in turn makes the facility safer for the client. The safety of clients is very important.

Some of the things that healthcare facilities have done to prevent errors and mistakes include:

- Creating a "No Blame" Workplace:
  Healthcare workers are not punished when they make a mistake. Employees are not asked, "Who did this?". Instead, they are asked, "What happened in this situation?" and "What can we do so that this never happens again?".

- Root Cause Analysis:
  This is a new way of investigating errors. It digs all the way down to the root cause of the problem, not the person. The root of the problem is most often a process or procedure that was unable to prevent the mistake. Processes and procedures that do not allow a healthcare worker to make a mistake are the best routines in healthcare. Processes and procedures that allow a worker to make a mistake are faulty; therefore, they must be improved and corrected so they do not permit any errors or mistakes. Once a problem-prone process is identified, it is corrected so future errors do not occur.

Basic Rules to Prevent Mistakes and Errors

- Be Competent:
  Do not do anything unless absolutely certain you can do it in the correct manner. If you are not sure of something, ask the nurse for help.

- Communicate Well:
  Keep open all lines of communication with your supervisor. Report all things that are not normal or are different for the patient and document all care. Documentation is a form of communication. Also, report to the supervisor all mistakes and safety concerns.

- Respond to Clients at All Times:
  Listen and respond to patients at all times. If a patient turns on his/her call light, respond immediately. If the alarm is something you can take care of, do so; however, if it is an IV alarm that you cannot work with as a CNA, call the nurse.

- Listen to Clients:
  If a patient has a question about a treatment, stop, check your assignment, and speak with the nurse.

- Identify Clients:
  Accurately identify the client each and every time you enter his/her room. Never skip this part of client care.

Falls

Falls are one of the biggest, and most costly, high-risk mistakes in healthcare facilities. All clients should be screened and assessed for falls risk when they are admitted; they must also be reassessed for falls whenever their condition changes. For example, a patient should be reassessed for falls when he/she returns to the floor after an operation.

If the client has been identified as at risk for falls, special preventive measures must be immediately implemented. Some of the risk factors that place patients at risk for falls include:
- Poor vision
- Age
- Confusion
- Slow reaction time
- Incontinence
- Some medications
- Some diseases and disorders
- Safety risks and hazards in the patient environment

People with a visual impairment and who cannot see well may trip over things they cannot see, particularly in a strange, new place such as a hospital. Patients should be given eyeglasses and encouraged to use them. The elderly do not react to dangers as quickly as younger people. For example, they may slip and fall when they cannot react quickly enough to avoid a puddle on the floor.

Confused people may not have good judgment, and they may be unaware of safety hazards. They may, for example, drink cleaning chemicals that are unsecured, and they may attempt to climb out a window.

Patients who are incontinent of urine and/or feces often slip on these wastes when trying to go to and from the bathroom. An infant may roll onto the floor from a table when left unattended, even for a moment; you must never leave alone an infant without holding onto him/her. The elderly and the very young are at greatest risk for falls.

Some medications, like sedation, make a patient sleepy and at risk for falls; patients may also fall because they have poor balance, weak balance, or poor coordination. Many older patients and those who have had a stroke have poor balance, and they ambulate with a poor gait—the lack of coordination and poor muscle control. The assistance of a physical therapist may be highly beneficial to these clients so they do not experience a fall. Likewise, some patients with other diseases and disorders, such as arthritis and Parkinson's disease, are also at risk for falls.

Shoes and slippers that are not skid proof are a danger in terms of slips and falls. All patients must have sturdy, skid-proof shoes or slippers that fit well. All wet floors must be clearly marked off. If there is a puddle on the floor, clean it up immediately or call housekeeping to clean it up if it is too large for you to handle. Lastly, environmental safety hazards such as high glare floors and clutter must be prevented and eliminated. Clutter in client rooms and hallways must never be present.

Preventing falls is a team effort. Special measures and special nursing care must start as soon as any patient or resident is assessed as a falls risk. For example, the patient may get a bed and chair alarm that will alert staff when he/she attempts to get out of the bed or chair. The nursing assistant must respond immediately to these alarms. The patient may also have other things such as padded briefs, a low bed, and a gym mat next to the bed to lessen the injury in case of a fall. The nursing assistant must ensure that all of these things are in place and in correct working order.

In the past, restraints were used to prevent falls. Now, restraints are the LAST resort to prevent falls and to prevent other things such as pulling out catheters and IV lines.

Restraints and Restraint Use

Doctors and some nurses must make a very difficult decision about when and how to restrain a person. In healthcare, the goal is to be "restraint free." We do not want to use restraints, but sometimes they are necessary when patients are in danger of severely hurting themselves and/or others. In the past, healthcare providers used to tie patients to their chairs and beds and raise the side rails to prevent patients from falling. This is no longer done. Restraints, including side rails, used to prevent a person from getting out of the bed are the last resort; many other preventive measures can be used to prevent falls.

Preventive or alternative measures prevent the use of restraints for many patients and residents. A restraint is used only when these preventive measures do not work and when the person is still in danger of hurting himself/herself or others. They are NEVER used to make healthcare workers' jobs easier. They are NOT for staff convenience. They are also NEVER used to punish a person. They are used only to protect a person from harm. A doctor's order is necessary before a restraint is used unless there is an extreme emergency; in this case, the registered nurse is able to initiate the use of restraints. In these situations, the registered nurse can initiate the use of restraints only for a brief period of time until the doctor can follow up with an order.

A restraint is anything that restricts a person from complete freedom to move about. Restraints can be physical or chemical. A chemical restraint is a medicine, or drug, that makes the person very sleepy and unable to move about freely. A physical restraint is any device placed on or near a person that stops him/her from moving about freely. Physical restraints include a vest, soft padded wrist restraints, side rails used to stop a person from getting out of bed, a sheet tied around a person to keep him/her from falling out of a chair, and a mitten to stop a person from pulling on his/her urinary catheter.

Restraints are most often used in hospitals and nursing homes to prevent falls; to stop a person from pulling out a necessary tube, line, or catheter such as an IV line or a urinary drainage catheter; and to protect patients, residents, family members, staff, and visitors from the violent actions of a patient.

When needed, several restraints can be used; however, the LEAST restrictive of all must be used. The restraint that keeps the person safest and takes away the LEAST amount of freedom is the one that should be used and ordered by the doctor. For example, if a client is tugging on an IV line on the left arm, a mitten restraint can be placed on the client's right hand to prevent this. Likewise, a vest, rather than four-point leather restraints, can be used to prevent combative behavior.

Follow exactly your hospital or nursing home procedure on how to apply a restraint. Do NOT do it in any other manner. You must follow the procedure without any changes.

Restraints should never be put on:
- An arm with an arterial line
- Skin that is burned, sore, or injured in any way
- A broken arm or leg

Restraints should never be tied to a part of a bed or chair that is moveable. For example, a vest restraint should NEVER be tied to a side rail or the bottom of the bed that moves when the head of the bed is moved up. Do NOT put a restraint on a patient or resident if you are unsure of the correct procedure. Do NOT care for a person with a restraint if you are unsure of the correct procedure. Ask the nurse for instructions.

All restrained patients or residents must be observed very often. At times, you may have to stay in the room with the patient or resident. Other times, you may be asked to observe the patient every 5, 10, or 15 minutes, depending on the patient or resident and his/her condition. If the person is stable and safe, the nurse may ask you to observe the person every hour or so.

Registered nurses (RN):
- Assess the patient or resident and his/her current condition
- Plan for and provide preventive actions that can keep the person safe without the use of restraints
- Begin restraints with a doctor's order and without a doctor's order in emergency situations
- Assign the care of patients who have a restraint

Nursing assistants:
- Provide care to patients with restraints
- Put on and take off restraints, as assigned
- Observe and report to the nurse the patient's condition and his/her responses to restraints

When monitoring the restrained patient or resident, watch the person and observe his/her:

- Response to the Restraint:
  Is the patient still in danger of harm with the restraint on? Has the person gotten better and perhaps no longer needs the restraint? Does it seem that the person is no longer confused and, therefore, not in need of a restraint to stop him/her from pulling out an IV, for example?

- Physical State:
  Is the person safe and not in danger of harm from the restraint? Is the person breathing normally? Is the skin color and circulation good? Is the restraint too tight or too loose? Is the person comfortable, clean, and dry? Does the client need any help from you?

- Mental Status:
  Is the person confused? Is the patient or resident angry, upset, or agitated? Is the person afraid or fearful?

All monitoring and care of a person with a restraint must be documented and reported to the nurse. Some hospitals and nursing homes use a restraint flow sheet. You must immediately report to the nurse if you notice something abnormal or incorrect while monitoring the person in restraints. If the person is in danger, fix the problem if you can. If you cannot fix the problem, call for help. Do NOT leave the person alone when he/she is in danger. Stay with the person and call for help.

Other things that can prevent the use of restraints, particularly for falls, include more frequent patient monitoring and observation; moving the patient closer to the nurse's station for closer observation; having a trained volunteer sitter or family member stay with the patient; keeping the patient's areas well-lit and safe; keeping a patient's urinal, commode, and personal possessions within close reach; keeping the nurse call bell within close reach; reminding the patient to call for help when he/she needs it; and always answering call lights immediately and without delay.

Patient Identification

Faulty and incomplete patient identification can lead to very serious and even deadly mistakes. Nursing assistants and other hospital personnel must accurately identify all patients before administering any care. By taking shortcuts and not correctly identifying patients, many different medical errors or mistakes can occur including the wrong patient undergoing surgery and the wrong patient's blood or urine sample going to the lab.

Examples of other errors and/or mistakes related to patient identification that can cause harm include a patient being diagnosed with a serious and terminal disease such as cancer because of a mislabeled laboratory specimen, a patient dying from being given too much insulin because a nursing assistant recorded the wrong patient's blood glucose level, a patient being sent to the wrong nursing home because the paperwork given to the transportation service was written incorrectly, and an infant getting circumcised against the wishes of his parents because the client's identity was not checked.

Patient identification errors tend to occur more often when the patient is blind, deaf, hard of hearing; or confused or has a mental problem, is sleepy or in a coma, or is under the influence of some medications and drugs; or when the patient is an infant or very young. Identity is also a challenge when patients in the nursing unit and in the facility have the same or similar names. For example, Thomas Smith can be confused with another client who has the name Thomas Smyth.

Pay extra attention to the client's identification. If you are unsure or have a feeling the client is not who he/she says he/she is or who you think he/she is, then double check. Check not only his/her identification band, but also his/her medical chart. It is always better to be safe than sorry, so check with your supervisor if all else fails to reassure you.

The following are ways to correctly identify patients:

- Most patients should be wearing a secure identification band; some patients may also have a photograph used for identification. Do not provide any patient with any type of care unless you are able to verify his/her identification by looking at his/her identification band or photo.

- The first and last name of the patient, including the spelling, should be checked and rechecked. If there are any differences, immediately consult with the nurse.

- Ask the patient for his/her first and last name. This verbal statement can help with some patients, but is not always helpful when the patient is confused, young, an

51

infant, or a person with a mental illness. Again, if there is any question about the patient's identification, check with the nurse about how to proceed.

- All treatment records must be compared to the patient's verified identification so the correct patient gets the correct treatment or procedure.

- If the patient questions you when you tell them what you are going to be doing with him/her, this could be a sign that he/she is not the correct patient. Check his/her identity again.

- Refer to the patient by name. This means that identifying them by a room number or illness is the incorrect way to identify the patient. For example, asking a member of the healthcare staff to "take the baby from room 16 to get his circumcision" can be misheard as perhaps room 15, which can lead to the procedure being done to the wrong patient. Likewise, referring to a client as "the stroke patient" leads to identity mistakes and is also disrespectful.

  Do not refer to patients by room numbers for any reason. Patients can be moved or even move themselves from room to room or from bed to bed. This can happen because a patient is confused or suffering from a form of dementia. A patient should always be identified by referring to his/her first and last name, date of birth, and other unique identifiers, NOT the room number or diagnosis.

- Check the patient's identification against the medical order(s). Be very careful when doing this, especially when there is more than one patient having the same procedure or when two or more patients have the same or similar names. For example, if Beatrice Smith and Betty Smith are both in the same unit of the facility, pay careful attention to the orders so that Betty Smith is not brought into the operating room instead of Beatrice Smith.

- While referring to the patient's identification band, carefully label his/her specimens, equipment, and supplies such as bedpans and urinals.

- Make suggestions if you think there is a problem or issue regarding your patient identification process.

  You can help. In this way, your facility can remain safe. Always report to the nurse or your supervisor anything you think can be improved.

Avoiding Distractions, Managing Stress, and Managing Time

Several mistakes occur when you are tired, distracted and/or interrupted, under a lot of stress, or in a hurry. These types of mistakes are less likely to occur if you make sure to:

- Get Plenty of Rest and Manage Your Time Properly:
  Getting at least eight hours of sleep every night ensures that you have gotten plenty of rest and that you won't be tired at work. A restful sleep is necessary in order to be alert at work.

- Focus:
  It is important to stay focused on the patients and their care at all times. Do not allow noises, television, or conversations to distract you. Focusing on the client you are caring for and on nothing else can prevent you from making mistakes.

- Double Check Your Assignment and New Things:
  When you are used to the same routine with your clients, you can sometimes forget something new that is ordered. For example, one of your clients may be scheduled for a procedure the next morning that requires an enema the night before. This is a new order, and because you are not used to giving that patient an enema at night, you may forget to do it.

  Also, when something has been discontinued for the patient, you may forget and continue to do it for the client. Always check your assignment and speak with the nurse if you are unsure what should, and should not, be done for the patient.

- Manage Your Stress:
  Stress is a reaction to life changes that upsets our balance. Stress can be caused by physical changes such as illness and mental changes such as anxiety and fear about caring for so many clients.

  Most people must deal with stress in everyday life in one way or another. Nursing assistants must also deal with stress. Stress can lead to errors and mistakes, so it must be managed properly. Some of the ways you can manage stress include:

  o Determine the source of the stress and try to eliminate it. If you cannot eliminate the source, try to change your thinking about it. For example, it is NOT a life-threatening stress when your bath water is not hot enough, so do not worry about it to the point where it endangers you, your inner peace, and your clients. Put it into perspective. It is NOT a major catastrophe.

  o Learn how to say no. Do not say yes when you cannot handle anymore. For example, if your church is looking for volunteers to help with child-care on Sundays, do not volunteer if you already have too much to do. This does not make you a bad person; it simply means you do not have time to volunteer.

  o Talk about your stress and stressors. Talking about your stress and venting your feelings are good ways to release stress. You can talk to a friend, family member, or even a therapist. If you are concerned or need to talk about something, reach out. Reaching out and getting help is not a weakness; it is a strength.

- o Set realistic goals, and do not put yourself in a position where you cannot handle or deal with multiple tasks and goals. Also, set priorities. All tasks cannot be done in one day. Decide which are most important and do these first so you do not get overwhelmed.

- o Exercise and eat a healthful diet.

Reporting All Safety Problems, Errors, and Mistakes

All errors, mistakes, "near misses," incidents, and accidents such as falls and burns must be immediately reported. These reports aim to prevent future errors, mistakes, and accidents. These reports give everyone the opportunity to understand why the mistakes were made and to determine how these problems can be eliminated in the future. The overall goal of reporting errors is to help make improvements and to prevent the errors from occurring in the future.

Protecting Patient Safety with Root Cause Analysis

Root cause analysis is the method used to analyze problems, errors, and mistakes in order to prevent them in the future. Mistakes occur because of weak procedures and processes, not people.

A root cause analysis team, which consists of people who usually perform the process being analyzed, is developed. For example, a root cause analysis team researching the problem of the wrong procedure or surgery on the wrong patient may consist of nursing assistants, who bring patients to the operating room, and operating room nurses and transport staff.

These teams use a variety of tools and techniques including discussing the error and the process, brainstorming, flow charting, fish bone diagrams, and careful thought. The process of root cause analysis can take several hours or even several days. The process is not complete until all team members are able to determine the root contributing factors and write a corrective plan of action to prevent future problems.

This plan is then implemented, and, hopefully, future errors and mistakes are prevented.

INTERNAL DISASTERS

Disasters affect several people every year. There are several types of disasters, but fire is perhaps the most common. Disasters such as floods, hurricanes, lightning, landslides, earthquakes, volcanoes, and wild fires are natural disasters. Some disasters can be chemical, while others can be related to acts of terror such as explosions, chemical attacks, and germ attacks.

All hospitals and other healthcare facilities have plans in place for all these emergencies.

Fires

In order for fires to start, there must be heat, air, and something to burn (fuel). Unless all three are present, a fire cannot start, so a way to prevent fires is to eliminate one of these necessities. For example, a fire can be prevented when an open flame (heat) is NOT allowed near oxygen (gas that burns) in a room filled with air. Fire can also be prevented when cigarette smoking (heat) is not permitted in client rooms or beds (something that burns). Other burnable items include solids such as paper and wood, liquids such as grease, gases such as gas fumes, and electricity.

Fire prevention includes facility-wide smoke detectors and fire sprinklers as well as established policies and procedures relating to smoking, oxygen use, electrical safety, and the use of other gases such as nitrous oxide. Facilities also have established policies and procedures to deal with fires, other internal disasters, and external disasters should they occur. All nursing assistants and other members of the facility must be fully knowledgeable about these procedures because when a disaster occurs there is no time to read the manual; immediate action is necessary.

You MUST act quickly if and when a fire starts. You must R-A-C-E.

- **R**escue everyone in danger; get all clients and visitors out of danger by following the fire plan set up by your facility.

- **A**larm; a fire alarm MUST be pulled.

- **C**onfine or contain the fire. Close all doors and windows; fire doors are supposed to automatically close to contain the fire in a small area and to prevent its spread to other areas of the facility.

- **E**xtinguish the fire only if it is safe to do so and if it is not possible to injure yourself or anyone else. When small fires are burning a solid such as paper, they can be put out with water or a fire extinguisher. If the fire is too large to handle, get out and wait for professional firefighters or your facility's fire squadron.

When a fire occurs, you may be instructed to evacuate patients. The two methods of evacuation are vertical and horizontal evacuation. When instructed to do a vertical evacuation, you will move patients from one floor to another. For example, when a fire starts on the fourth floor, you will be instructed to move clients to a lower level because smoke and fire spread upward. When instructed to do a horizontal evacuation, you will move patients from one area of the floor to another on the same floor as far away as possible from the fire.

All medical facilities must have emergency evacuation plans, and they should be posted so they can be referred to, and followed, in a rapid manner. Elevators are never used during a fire emergency. Elevators are reserved for firefighters and other emergency personnel and can lose electricity and trap people inside during a fire. The stairway is the only path of exit that can be used. For obvious reasons, many patients will need assistance during vertical evacuations.

If a fire is blocking a client's exit from his/her room, the door should be shut to keep out the fire and a towel or blanket placed at the bottom of the door to keep out the smoke.

If a fire alarm sounds when you and/or your patient are in the room with the door closed, feel the door BEFORE opening it. A hot door means the fire is just on the other side of it, so leave the door closed. Do NOT open it; instead, put a towel or blanket at the bottom of the door to keep out the smoke and call for help.

Nursing assistants should practice fire drills often to ensure they know and are able to follow the fire plan and escape. Practice makes perfect. Practice saves lives.

Fire Extinguishers

All medical facilities must have fire extinguishers. There are several different types of fire extinguishers, which include:

Type A: This extinguisher can be used to put out fires only on common solids such as paper, wood, and cloth. It CANNOT be used on oil, grease, or electrical fires.

Type B: This extinguisher is used to put out fires on liquids and gases such as gasoline, oil, and grease. It can be used on kitchen grease and fat fires. It CANNOT be used on electrical fires.

Type C: This extinguisher is used to put out electrical fires.

Type AB: This extinguisher is a combination of a type A and type B fire extinguisher. It can be used on solids such as paper, wood, and cloth (like the A type) and on liquid and gas fires including kitchen grease and fat fires (like the B type).

Type BC: Similar to the type AB fire extinguisher, the type BC fire extinguisher is a combination of a type B and type C fire extinguisher. The type BC can be used on electrical, liquid, and gas fires (like the B and C types).

Type ABC: This extinguisher is the BEST of all; it puts out all kinds and types of fires. It is highly recommended that these be in every healthcare facility and in the home. They can be purchased at almost every home improvement store for very little money.

It is required that all fire extinguishers be checked regularly to ensure they are fully charged and ready to use in an emergency.

To use a fire extinguisher, employ the P-A-S-S method:

- **Pull** the pin.

- Aim at the base, or bottom, of the fire or flame.
- Squeeze the trigger while holding the extinguisher straight up.
- Sweep, or move the spray, from side to side to completely cover the fire.

Smoke

If a room fills with smoke, the rule is to GET LOW AND GO. Smoke will fill a room from the ceiling down. Clients and visitors MUST get to the floor and crawl. As mentioned earlier, the door should be felt for heat, and, if it is safe to exit the room, everyone should cover his/her nose and mouth with a wet rag and crawl out of the area and out of danger.

What to Do When a Client's Clothes Are on Fire

The rule for this disaster is to STOP, DROP, AND ROLL. Tell the client, or any other person, to STOP and DROP, NOT run. Running will add air to the fire and make it more serious. Tell the person to lie down on the floor and cover his/her face with the hands; then roll him/her over and over again to smother the flames. The nursing assistant should also cover the person with a blanket or another item to put out the flames and smother the fire. Do NOT fan a fire with your hands. This, like running, will only worsen the fire.

Tornados and Serious Hurricanes

The following steps must be taken in case of a tornado:

- Go to the lowest level of the building near the center of an interior room that has no windows, doors, or outside walls. Do NOT open windows. Quickly close them if you can. These measures protect people from flying debris.

- Evacuate if told to do so. Close all interior doors.

- Keep curtains and blinds closed.

- Cover your face and head with your arms and crouch down.

- If you become trapped under fallen objects, cover your mouth with a handkerchief or clothing to keep out dust.

Terrorism

Terrorism, such as what happened with the World Trade Center, is described as the use of violence and force against people and property. There are several different types of terrorism such as chemical, biological, nuclear, and radiological weapons, all of which can lead to serious health problems and dcath.

If an act of terrorism occurs in your facility, follow the facility's instructions because responses to these acts vary greatly in terms of the type and severity of the act. For example, after a telephone bomb threat has been received, you may simply be advised to be aware of your surroundings and to stay in place while the security team or police search for a bomb.

Preventing Back Injuries

It is far easier to prevent a back injury than it is to live with a bad back. Fortunately, many things can help prevent back injuries. Some are done by the person off the job, some are done by the healthcare worker on the job, and others are done by the hospital or nursing home.

Some of the things you can do at home to prevent back injuries include:

- Exercise:
  Exercise regularly by swimming, running, jogging, walking, or rowing or complete muscle strengthening or stretching exercises.

- Rest:
  Get enough sleep and rest.

- Good Diet:
  A good diet helps keep a body healthy, strong, and in good shape.

- Healthful Body Weight:
  Excess body weight puts extra strain on your back and stomach muscles.

- Good Posture:
  You can prevent back pain and back problems by using good posture while sitting, standing, and lifting.

One of the most important things you can do to prevent hurting your back at work is to GET HELP when you need it. Also, use a mechanical lifting device whenever possible.

In order to prevent backache, use the following steps when lifting, moving, transporting, or doing any other physical activity:

1. Explain to the person what you are about to do. Even very weak patients can help you with a lift or transfer when he/she knows what you are about to do.

2. Stretch and warm up if your body is not warm and loose. Shake out your body. Stretch your arms up toward the ceiling. Jog in place for a couple of seconds.

3. Stay as close as possible to the person or object you are about to lift.

4. Face the person or object you are about to lift.

5. Keep your back straight up and down.

6. Tuck in your chin and keep your neck and head straight up and down.

7. Keep your feet wide apart so you have a wide base of support.

8. Pivot on your feet in the direction of the move. For example, if pulling up a person in bed with the help of another person, remain facing the person during the lift, but shift your weight by rocking onto the foot closest to the head of the bed. If moving a person from a bed to a chair, stand with your feet wide apart and pivot from facing the bed to facing the chair, in the direction of the move. Do NOT twist. Pivot and keep your spine, or back, straight.

9. Ensure you have a good grip on the object you are about to lift.

10. Use the long and strong muscles of your legs to lift. Do NOT use the muscles of your back to lift. For example, if you are lifting a scale off the floor, bend at the knees and squat down. Do NOT bend your back. After you grip the scale, raise your body to a straight position with the scale as close as possible to your body. Reverse these steps to put down the scale on the floor.

11. Use smooth and slow motions. Do NOT hurry; take your time. Do not use jerky motions; they can hurt your back.

12. Take small breaks between lifts. Take a deep breath and rest for a moment.

13. Another basic back safety rule is to PUSH, NOT PULL. Pushing is much safer than pulling.

For the last several years, many hospitals and other companies have used back belts and back supports to protect workers' backs against injury. These back supports, seen in home improvement stores, are a matter of choice. Some people think these back belts help prevent back injuries; others do not know if they do. Nonetheless, if you are given a back belt to use as you work, wear it. Wear it properly, but do not think you do not need to use good body mechanics and lifting skills. These skills must be used with and without a back belt.

THERAPEUTIC/TECHNICAL PROCEDURES

Vital Signs

Vital signs include assessing body temperature, pulse, blood pressure, and respiratory rate.

Body Temperature:
Body temperature is the difference between the amount of heat produced and the amount of heat lost. When taken orally, a normal body temperature is 98.6° F, which is 36.7° to 37° C. When a patient's temperature exceeds 98.6°, the patient has a fever, which is a sign of infection. A higher than normal temperature is called hyperthermia. When a person has a temperature below 98.6°, it is called hypothermia. Hypothermia can occur when a person is exposed to the cold. High and low temperatures must be reported to the nurse because these temperatures are not normal.

Body temperature can be taken different ways: in the person's mouth, under the tongue, in the rectum, in the ear, or under the arm pit or axillae.

Body temperature is usually taken orally, except when the client is an infant, a young child, a person with a rectal problem, or a patient who is unconscious or uncooperative. Other routes are preferable for these patients. For infants and young children, the best way to take temperature is in the ear. Other clients, except for those with heart disease, a seizure disorder, or a rectal disorder, can have their temperature taken rectally or by using an electronic thermometer that takes the temperature in the ear.

Pulses:
Pulse is the number of beats per minute that the heart beats or contracts. There are different areas where a patient's pulse can be felt or heard. For example, you can hear, or auscultate, the apical pulse by using a stethoscope over the center region of the chest and listening to the heart beat. You can also use your index and middle fingers to feel the patient's pulse over the radius near the wrist, on the side of the head in the temporal area, on the neck to feel the carotid pulse, in the groin for the femoral pulse, on the front of the foot for the dorsalis pedis pulse, behind the knee for the popliteal pulse, and near the ankle for the posterior tibial pulse.

Most pulses are counted by using the fingers to feel the heart beat on the wrist to get the radial pulse. The normal pulse is regular and normally is between 80 and 100 beats per minute for adults. If the pulse is less than 80 beats per minute, it is slow and is called bradycardia; if the pulse is more than 100 beats per minute, the pulse is considered fast and more rapid than normal. This is called tachycardia. It is not normal to hear or feel an irregular pulse. If the patient has a slow pulse (bradycardia), a rapid pulse (tachycardia) or an irregular pulse, report it to the nurse because these are not normal findings.

Blood Pressure:
Blood pressure results from the heart's pumping and resting actions and activity. The upper number of the blood pressure indicates the amount of pressure that occurs when the heart is pumping. This number is called systole, or the systolic blood pressure. The lower number of the blood pressure indicates the amount of pressure when the heart is resting. This number is called diastole, or the diastolic blood pressure. The diastolic blood pressure is less than the systolic blood pressure. For example, when a patient has a blood pressure of 156/87, the diastolic blood pressure is 87, and the systolic blood pressure is 156.

The normal blood pressure for an adult should be about 120/80 with a systolic blood pressure of 120 and a diastolic blood pressure of 80. When the blood pressure is low, it is referred to as hypotension, or low blood pressure. When the blood pressure is high, it is referred to as hypertension. Hypotension can be related to a number of different problems including bleeding and hemorrhage; hypertension can result from heart disease and other health problems.

A client's blood pressure reading is most commonly taken on the upper arm just above the elbow, but it can also be taken in other sites on the body such as the legs. When checking blood pressure, use a stethoscope and follow these steps:

1. To get an accurate blood pressure reading, allow the person to rest quietly for about five minutes if he/she has just engaged in physical activity.

2. Place the cuff on the upper portion of the arm. Tighten the cuff so only one finger can be slipped under it. Ensure that the measurement valve is visible on the inside of the arm. Check to see if the valve is closed on the cuff; turn the screw clockwise until tight.

3. Manually locate the brachial pulse using your index and middle fingers.

4. Put the stethoscope earpieces into your ears. Place the stethoscope's diaphragm on the brachial artery.

5. Begin pumping the cuff until the meter reads about 150 mmHg. Slowly turn the valve to gradually release the air.

6. Listen for the first sound and read the number shown at that point. Record the number as the systolic pressure. Continue to listen for when the sound changes or drops off. Record this number as the diastolic pressure.

7. Record the client's blood pressure, like you do for other vital signs, and also record the date and the precise time it was taken.

In addition to documenting, all abnormal findings must also be reported to the nurse. Many healthcare agencies and hospitals now use automatic blood pressure and pulse measurement machines.

Respirations:
Respiratory rates are the most consciously controlled of all vital signs. Respirations are the number of breaths a patient takes each minute. The normal respiratory rate is 18 to 22 per minute, but it can be lower when the patient is sleeping and higher when the patient is exercising.

A high respiratory rate is called tachypnea, a slow respiratory rate is called hypopnea, and a lack of any respirations is called apnea.

Emergency Resuscitation

Cardiopulmonary resuscitation (CPR) is a two-part method used in healthcare facilities and the community to save lives. The two parts of cardiopulmonary resuscitation are:

- Compressions:
  This first part of CPR involves pressing on the person's chest. This gives the person's body the blood flow necessary to survive when the heart has stopped and is no longer pumping blood to the body and vital organs, including the brain.

- Rescue Breathing:
  This second part is breathing. This gives the person the oxygen necessary to live when he/she can no longer breathe on his/her own. In the past, mouth-to-mouth breathing was administered, but now, with standard precautions, a special one-way valve mask is used.

Keeping oxygen flowing into the brain and heart is the most essential component of this procedure. If CPR is done quickly enough, the heart and brain can recover, but if the heart stops and CPR is not given, the brain and the person will die within a couple of minutes. CPR saves thousands of lives every year. It is twice more likely for a person to live if CPR is given than if it isn't given.

The number one most common type of death among adults occurs when the heart stops beating. The most common reason for this is heart disease, and heart disease is commonly seen in the elderly. The elderly are often cared for in hospitals and other healthcare facilities, including home healthcare, so it is quite important that people who work in these places know how to perform CPR.

Contrastingly, infants are most often affected with respiratory arrest, after which the heart stops beating.

C-A-B
The American Heart Association's CAB, which stands for **C**irculation **A**irway **B**reathing, helps people remember the order in which to perform the steps of CPR.

- **C**irculation: Restore blood circulation with chest compressions
  1. Put the person on his/her back on a firm surface.
  2. Kneel next to the person's neck and shoulders.
  3. Place the heel of one hand over the center of the person's chest, between the nipples. Place your other hand on top of the first hand. Keep your elbows straight and position your shoulders directly above your hands.
  4. Use your upper body weight, not just your arms, as you push straight down on the chest at least two inches. Push hard at a rate of about 100 compressions a minute.

- **A**irway: Clear the airway
  1. After you have performed 30 chest compressions at the rate of 100 compressions per minute, open the person's airway using the head-tilt, chin-lift maneuver. Put your palm on the person's forehead and gently tilt the head back. Then, with the other hand, gently lift the chin forward to open the airway.
  2. Check for normal breathing for about five or 10 seconds. Look for chest motion, listen for normal breath sounds, and feel for the person's breath on your cheek and ear. If the person isn't breathing normally, begin rescue breathing.

- **B**reathing: Breathe for the person
  1. With the airway open (using the head-tilt, chin-lift maneuver), pinch the nostrils shut, make a seal, and using the special mask or Ambu bag, begin the breaths.
  2. Give the first rescue breath for about one second and check if the chest rises during this breath. If it does, give the second breath. If it does not, repeat the head-tilt, chin-lift maneuver and give another breath. The chest will not rise with rescue breathing when the airway is not completely opened by the rescuer or when there is an obstruction in the airway. When the chest rises, perform 30 chest compressions followed by two rescue breaths. These 30 chest compressions and two rescue breaths are considered one cycle.
  3. Resume chest compressions to restore circulation.
  4. Continue CPR until there are signs of movement or emergency medical personnel take over.

Adult CPR (8 years of age or older)
Before starting CPR, check:
- Is the person conscious or unconscious?
- If the person appears unconscious, tap or shake his/her shoulder and ask loudly, "Are you ok?"
- If the person doesn't respond and two people are available, one should call for help, and one should begin CPR. If you are alone and have immediate access to a telephone, call for help before beginning CPR unless you think the person has become unresponsive because of suffocation such as from drowning. In this special case, begin CPR for one minute and then call for help.
- If an automatic defibrillator is immediately available, deliver one shock if instructed to do so by the device and then begin CPR.

Pediatric CPR (1 year of age to 8 years of age)
- The procedure for giving CPR to a child 1 to 8 years of age is essentially the same as that for an adult, with the following differences.
- If you're alone, perform five cycles of compressions and breaths on the child, which should take about two minutes, and then call for help.
- Use only one hand to perform heart compressions.
- Breathe more gently.

- Use the same compression-breath rate as used for adults: 30 compressions followed by two breaths for each cycle. Following the two breaths, immediately begin the next cycle of compressions and breaths.

Infant CPR

Most arrests in babies are respiratory arrests that occur with sudden infant death, drowning, and choking. If you know the baby has an airway obstruction, perform first aid for choking. If you don't know why the baby isn't breathing, perform CPR.

To begin, examine the situation. Stroke the baby and watch for a response such as movement, but don't shake him/her.

If there's no response, follow the CAB procedures below and time the call for help as follows:
- If you're the only rescuer and CPR is needed, do CPR for two minutes — about five cycles — before calling for help or your local emergency number.
- If another person is available, have him/her call for help immediately while you attend to the baby.

Circulation: Restore blood circulation
1. Place the baby on his/her back on a firm, flat surface such as a table. The floor or ground also will suffice.
2. Imagine a horizontal line drawn between the baby's nipples. Place two fingers of one hand just below this line, in the center of the chest.
3. Gently compress the chest about 1.5 inches.
4. Count aloud as you pump in a fairly rapid rhythm. You should pump at a rate of 100 compressions a minute.

Airway: Clear the airway
1. After 30 compressions, gently tip the head back by lifting the chin with one hand and pushing down on the forehead with the other hand.
2. In no more than 10 seconds, put your ear near the baby's mouth and check for breathing: look for chest motion, listen for breath sounds, and feel for breath on your cheek and ear.

Breathing: Breathe for the infant
1. Cover the baby's mouth and nose with your mouth.
2. Prepare to give two rescue breaths. Use the strength of your cheeks to deliver gentle puffs of air, instead of deep breaths from your lungs, to slowly breathe into the baby's mouth one time, taking one second for the breath. Watch to see if the baby's chest rises. If it does, give a second rescue breath. If it doesn't, repeat the head-tilt, chin-lift maneuver and then give the second breath.
3. If the baby's chest still doesn't rise, examine the mouth to make sure no foreign material is inside. If you see the object, sweep it out with your finger. If the airway seems blocked, perform first aid for a choking baby.
4. Give two breaths after every 30 chest compressions.

5. Perform CPR for about two minutes before calling for help unless someone else can make the call while you attend to the baby.
6. Continue CPR until you see signs of life or until medical personnel arrive.

How to Care for a Conscious Person Who is Choking

If you're present when someone is choking, act fast before he/she loses consciousness. There are only a few minutes from the time someone starts choking in which to save his/her life.

Look for Choking Signs:
The person may be holding the throat with both hands or making a high-pitched wheezing noise as he/she gasps for air. A conscious choking victim definitely won't be able to talk or breathe properly, and coughing will also be impossible.

Get the Choking Victim to Stand Up:
Once you have determined that you are, in fact, dealing with a conscious choking victim, treat the situation as an emergency and act quickly. Get someone else to call for professional help. Have the person stand up and position yourself directly behind him/her to perform the Heimlich maneuver to dislodge the obstruction, which is most often a piece of food.

Get Hands into Position:
Bring your arms around the person, making a fist with one of your hands, and then grab the wrist of that hand with your other hand. Place your fist just below the rib cage so that the thumb of your hand that is in a fist is sitting near the belly button. Then, thrust your fist inwards and up into the choking victim's chest. This should be a quick, deliberate motion. Don't worry about hurting the victim or bruising ribs.

Continue to make these thrusting movements quickly, in rapid succession, for as long as required to dislodge the obstruction.

Managing Behavior

Many older people have a behavior problem because they are confused with delirium or dementia; younger people may act poorly because they have a mental illness or delirium, confusion, or dementia after a head injury.

Delirium comes on, or appears, very fast and quickly. The person can be disoriented and confused. He/she may not be able to sleep. Some may see or hear things that are not really there. They may hear the voices of people who have died. They may see someone giving poison to another patient. This person may do dangerous things or become very fearful. He/she can react to this fear with dangerous or violent behavior.

Dementia is different from delirium. It comes on slowly. The person becomes more and more disoriented or confused in a slow way. The person's behavior can get worse and worse as time goes on. Alzheimer's disease is the most frequently seen dementia. Other diseases, such as Parkinson's disease, and an infection can also cause dementia.

Problematic behavior can be:

- Disruptive:
  These behaviors can upset other patients and residents and make them angry. Screaming, yelling, and cursing are examples of disruptive, disturbed patient behavior. Saying the same thing over and over and resisting, or fighting, nursing care are some other examples of this kind of behavior.

- Dangerous:
  These behaviors can hurt the person who commits them and also hurt others. This person can hurt others when he/she hits, kicks, bites, spits, or throws things. This person can hurt himself/herself by wandering outside of the healthcare facility.

A person can react to many things by using poor behaviors. He/she may hit a person if he/she is cold. The person may slap the nursing assistant if another person makes him/her upset. He/she may yell if the patient-care area or dining room is noisy. Things that can lead to poor behavior are called triggers. Triggers can be different to different people. Know your patients and what triggers them. Triggers can be:

- Physical:
  Patients may act out when they are in pain, soiled, tired, sick, thirsty, and hungry. Others react when they are constipated or are unable to see or hear what is going on around them.

- Environmental:
  Noise, too much or too little light, and an uncomfortable room temperature can be triggers. Nursing assistants and others should keep the patient-care area quiet and calm. It should be well-lit, and the temperature should be comfortable for clients.

- Related to Care Given:
  Bathing, getting out of bed, eating, dressing, and other things can trigger poor behavior. These triggers can be prevented if we give the person choices and complete tasks in small steps. Reward the patient with smiles and praise. If he/she resists, stop the task and try again later. This empathy and understanding prevents poor behaviors.

- Communication:
  Behaviors may be triggered if the person can't tell you what he/she wants or needs or can't talk to other patients and residents, family, or his/her doctor. Spend time with the patient. Listen to him/her closely. Use the person's name. Be calm. Do NOT argue with a patient or resident. Sit with the person. Talk to him/her slowly and at eye level. Do NOT stand while the person is sitting.

Preventing poor behavior and managing disturbed behavior requires a team effort. Sometimes, the patient may get medications and psychological help to prevent disturbed behavior. However, most patients can be managed with a team that prevents poor behavior. The nursing assistant is a very important member of the team's effort. Everyone must report and communicate patient changes. Everyone must follow the plan of care. Everyone must prevent and manage disturbed behavior.

Nursing assistants must know their patients and the triggers that lead to poor behavior. Try to calm a patient during care. Keep things the same and simple to prevent poor behavior. Know the best routine for the person and stick to it. Eliminate all physical, emotional, environmental, communication, and care triggers. Meet the person's needs so he/she does NOT react with disturbed behavior. Give simple instructions and repeat instructions, if needed. Listen to the patient so he/she can make known his/her needs; spend time with your patient and let him/her ask questions and tell you about his/her feelings.

Observe your patients and how they act with others. If a patient annoys another patient, encourage both to go to a different place. Approach a very confused patient from the side and speak face to face. Speak slowly, calmly, and use simple words. Ask simple 'yes' or 'no' questions. NEVER argue with the person even when he/she is wrong. Try to distract the person to a new or different thought.

Keep the patient-care area simple. Keep schedules and routines the same for people who act out when things are changed. Limit choices, if needed, and keep stress low. Encourage sleep by keeping a regular bed time and providing a quiet environment. Exercise, relaxation, pet therapy, music therapy, and socialization or exercise groups can lower stress and prevent poor behaviors.

Manage disruptive, unacceptable, or dangerous behaviors when they occur by staying calm, speaking softly, and showing respect; stop the task you are doing and call for help, if needed.

Nursing assistants immediately report and document all disruptive behavior. Tell the nurse, and document, what triggered the behavior, what happened, when it happened, where it happened, how long the behavior lasted, and what you did to stop the poor and dangerous behavior.

Skin Care and Preventing Pressure Ulcers

The reasons people get pressure ulcers include:

- Old Age:
  The normal aging process changes the skin and blood circulation. The skin can be dry, very fragile, easily irritated, and easily broken. Older people may also have poor circulation to the skin so the oxygen to the skin is insufficient to keep the skin healthy and without injury.

- Lack of Mobility:
  Pressure ulcers can occur from the pressure exerted when a person stays in the bed, chair, or wheelchair for a long time. Blood and oxygen is cut off to areas where bones are close to the skin, particularly the sacrum, elbows, ears, shoulders, toes, and heels, depending on the position in which the patient remains. Some of these bony areas can break down when a person is kept in one position for a long period of time.

- Poor Nutrition and Diet:
  Good nutrition, especially protein, and adequate fluids are needed for healthy skin.

- Presence of Moisture:
  Patients who are incontinent of urine or stool, who sweat a lot, and who have draining wounds are at risk for pressure ulcers. Moisture softens the skin so that it breaks.

- Mental, Neurological, and Other Physical Problems:
  When a patient is confused, very sleepy, in a coma, or paralyzed, he/she may not turn when sleeping so he/she will stay in one position for a long time unless turned and positioned by the nursing assistant.

- Friction and Shearing Forces:
  These forces occur when a patient is pulled up in bed or the chair. These forces can irritate and tear the skin.

- Foreign Bodies in the Bed or Chair:
  Uneven pressure is created when sheets are wrinkled and/or when items such as spoons, tissue boxes, eye glasses, food crumbs, hair pins, and other hard objects are left in the bed or chair because they cause pressure and pressure ulcers.

Warning Signs

A warning sign of a pressure ulcer is when pink skin on a bony area turns white. This white color occurs because red-colored blood in the area is cut off with pressure. Later, the skin will then become red, irritated, and warm. When the pressure continues, the top layers of the skin will break away, and an open sore will appear. It may get worse until all the skin layers are broken down and the bone, muscle, and joint are seen. The worst pressure ulcers affect the bones themselves.

The Prevention of Pressure Ulcers

Pressure ulcers can be prevented with proper skin care and by keeping patients clean and dry, looking at the patient and his/her skin, giving patients a good diet and plenty of fluids, helping patients walk, and turning and positioning patients often.

Turning and Positioning

There are several positions in which people can be placed while in the bed, unless the doctor says they cannot be in a certain position. Some of these positions are:

- Fowler's Position:
  The person is sitting straight up in the bed. The legs may be straight or bent a bit. This position is sometimes called the High Fowler's position.
  - Pressure Points: The heels, pelvis, spine and sacrum

- Semi-Fowlers Position:
  The person is sitting, but the angle of the bed is lower and not straight up. This position is sometimes called the Low Fowler's position.
  - Pressure Points: The heels, pelvis, spine and sacrum

- Supine or Back Lying Position:
  The person is lying flat on his/her back.
  - Pressure Points: The heels, sacrum, elbows, scapulae, and back of the head

- Prone Position:
  The person is lying on his/her stomach with the head turned to one side.
  - Pressure Points: The ankle bone area, knees, hip bone, shoulder, side of the head, and ears

- Lateral or Side Lying Position:
  The person is lying on his/her right or left hip.
  - Pressure Points: The toes, knees, male genitals, breasts, shoulder, cheek, and ears

- Sim's or Half Lateral and Half Prone Position:
  The person is lying in a half prone and half lateral position.
  - Pressure Points: The ears, cheek, shoulder, hip, feet, and toes

All of these positions lead to pressure on one or more parts of the body; therefore, the person must be repositioned at least every two hours.

If the client is limited to the bed or if he/she must spend a lot of time in bed, a certain type of mattress can help prevent pressure sores. The mattress automatically inflates and deflates length-wise and provides different pressure settings. The mattress will automatically turn the client from side to side every few minutes. This movement is not limited to the mattress; the entire bed rotates.

END OF LIFE CARE

The end of life requires special nursing care. All patients and family members at the end of life need good communication, physical comfort, emotional comfort, and spiritual comfort.

Nursing assistants play a very important role in end of life care. They observe and report all end of life needs to the charge nurse. They also provide end of life care. For example, a nursing assistant must report when a patient would like to see a minister so that the minister can visit with the dying patient. Nursing assistants may also be asked by the nurse to sit and talk to a resident so the resident will not fear being alone. Nursing assistants also must care for the family. They allow families to spend time with loved one, provide privacy, and make the family comfortable.

Nursing assistants communicate with patients who are in a coma or are unconscious. Hearing is the last sense to stop functioning at the end of life. Nursing assistants also observe and report signs of pain and distress. They provide a quiet room; a backrub; soothing music; physical care such as a bath, turning and positioning, and mouth care; a clean bed; and a clean room.

Post-Mortem Care

It is important that the client's loved ones are encouraged to grieve the loss of their friend or family member and to spend time with him/her to say goodbye.

Nursing assistants provide post-mortem care with dignity and respect for the person who has died. Each facility has its own steps for post-mortem care. In most cases, however, post-mortem care includes cleaning the client's body and preparing it for the funeral home. While nursing assistants do not apply make-up or position for a funeral, they do give the final bath and dress the body. All of this care is the same as if the client were still alive.

The final care of the client begins with giving him/her a bath, just as would be done if the client were alive. Something not always discussed in training about post-mortem care is the unexpected sounds or actions of the human body. Unexpected reflexes include eyes opening, a moan-like sound as the last bit of air in the lungs escapes during movement, and a final breath. Another important thing to remember is that as muscles relax to let air escape, so do muscles holding in other things.

Legal and Ethical Issues at the End of Life

At the end of life, all patients still have a right to dignity, the right to make decisions, the right to refuse treatments, and the right to privacy and confidentiality.

Some legal issues at the end of life include a living will, or advance directives, and a healthcare proxy.

Patients and residents across the country are encouraged to write which treatments they do and do NOT want at the end of life. These are put in a "living will" or "advance directives." This legal document is used to make decisions about whether or not to give a treatment or use a technology, such as tube feeding and a mechanical ventilator, when the patient is no longer able to give consent. Advance directives are legal documents that must be followed without exception.

A healthcare proxy is the legal appointment of a healthcare decision-making surrogate to the patient to make healthcare decisions for him/her, and in his/her best interest, when a situation occurs that was NOT already anticipated in the living will. Again, this document is legally and ethically binding.

DATA COLLECTION AND REPORTING

Nursing assistants and other healthcare workers are responsible for collecting, documenting, and reporting data. All documentation must be complete, correct, on time, legally correct, and professional. Most hospital and other healthcare facilities use computerized documentation, others may still use forms and papers to document, and others still may use a combination of the two. It is important to follow your facility's rules and regulations.

Two of the most important aspects of care that nursing assistants perform are observation and reporting. Observation is done by seeing, hearing, smelling, and feeling. For example, you may smell a strange and unusual mouth odor, or you may hear the patient crying. You collect data and information when you observe a patient.

Kinds of Data

Data can be either primary or secondary. Primary data is provided by the client himself/herself; secondary data is collected from other sources such as previous nursing notes and laboratory test results. An example of primary data is the patient's vital signs.

Data can also be classified as subjective or objective. Subjective data is not measurable or observable, and it typically consists of the client's own words. A statement from the client about his/her pain is subjective data. Contrastingly, objective data is measurable and observable. Vital signs are objective data. An example of subjective data is when the client states, "I have a headache." An example of objective data is feeling moisture and sweating on the patient's skin.

Lastly, data can be quantitative or qualitative. Quantitative data consists of numbers; qualitative data consists of words. The person's blood glucose level is quantitative data because it consists of numbers. The client's beliefs and statements about pain are subjective, qualitative data.

All data the nursing assistant collects must be documented, and all data that is abnormal or unusual for the patient must also be immediately reported to the nurse. For example, when the patient's temperature is 98.7° F, simply document it, but when it is 100.8° F, document and report it.

Documentation

Documentation is one of the most commonly used forms of communication in healthcare. Everything must be documented so all members of the healthcare team know what is happening in terms of the patient's status and care.

This documentation includes everything you do and observe. If you do not document something, it is considered not done; therefore, you must take the time to document anything and everything you have done. The many aspects of care that nursing assistants do, and document, include baths, showers, back care, turning and positioning, activities such as walking and range of motion exercises (if done), oral care, foot care, urinary catheter care, meal intake, and fluid intake.

The observations that nursing assistants must document include vital signs; meal intake; fluid intake; blood glucose readings (if you can take them); color of the skin; level of consciousness; orientation to time, place, and person; urinary drainage bag output; what the patient says; and behaviors such as anger and yelling.

All documentation must be complete and correct. You are responsible for writing what you do, see, hear, and feel. If you bathe a client at 9:15 a.m., you are responsible for documenting it. Do not write 9 a.m. or 9:30 a.m.; write that you bathed the client at 9:15 a.m. The same is true for all tasks. All documentation must be correct.

Each individual is responsible for his/her own documentation. Never ask anyone to document anything for you and never document anything for another person.

You are responsible for facts; all documentation should be objective facts, not opinions. Writing, "The client is uncooperative today." is incorrect because it is not something you did, saw, heard, or felt. You may have observed that the client refused to bathe, but you cannot assume that he/she is uncooperative or lazy. However, you can, and should, document, "The patient refused his/her bath."

Documentation also must be done in a timely fashion. Never wait until the end of your shift to document something. The documented information is extremely important. It is used by all members of the healthcare team.

For example, if you observe that a client is unsteady on his/her feet and/or tells you that he/she is feeling dizzy, document it as soon as possible. If you fail to document this information, or put it off for a period of time, another member of the healthcare team may try to ambulate the client, unaware of the difficulty. This can lead to a risk of the client falling.

All clients' medical records are legal documents. You can ensure your documentation is legal by writing only facts, not charting before something is done, not using abbreviations considered unacceptable, using blue or black ink unless using a computer, writing clearly, dating all notes, indicating the time you write the note, signing your full name and title (CNA), not scribbling out words after a mistake, and not using "white out" or anything else that covers up writing.

All documentation should be written in a professional manner. It is important to write clearly and legibly so the documentation can be read without problems. Spelling is also important. If you are unsure of how to spell a word, look it up. These are patient records, not a place for you to vent your feelings. For example, never write, "The physician didn't arrive to speak to the client until 11 a.m., although he told the client he would be there first thing in the morning." These types of statements reflect matters that should be privately discussed with your supervisor, not documented in the client's file.

Chapter 3: Physical Care Skills—Restorative Skills

PREVENTION

Much of a nurse assistant's work involves preventing complications and restoring function. For example, nursing assistants prevent pressure ulcers, the loss of muscle function, and other hazards of immobility by using techniques such as range of motion exercises, ambulation assistance, and out-of-bed activity.

The old adage, "Take an aspirin and go to bed." could not be further from good advice. Immobility leads to severe consequences in terms of many bodily functions and structures. These hazards are described below.

- The Musculoskeletal System:
  Some adverse musculoskeletal system effects of immobility include muscle weakness, muscular atrophy, contractures, stiff and painful joints, and disuse osteoporosis or arthritis.

- The Respiratory System:
  Some adverse respiratory system effects relating to immobility include hypostatic pneumonia as the result of pooled respiratory secretions, atelectasis that is also the result of pooled secretions in the bronchiole, decreased respiratory movement, decreased vital capacity, and shallow respirations.

- The Circulatory System:
  Some of the physiological changes that occur as the result of immobility include diminished cardiac reserve; orthostatic hypotension, which can place the person at risk for falls; venous stasis and venous vasodilation, which can lead to the formation of emboli; dependent edema; thrombophlebitis; and increased use of the Valsalva maneuver.

- The Urinary System:
  The urinary system can be affected by urinary stasis; renal stones, or calculi; urinary retention; urinary incontinence; and urinary tract infections.

- The Integumentary System:
  Immobility places clients at risk for skin breakdown, pressure ulcers, and poor skin turgor.

- The Metabolic System:
  Some of the complications of immobility relating to the metabolic system include diminished metabolic rate, negative nitrogen balance caused by increased catabolic protein breakdown, anorexia, and negative calcium balance caused by loss of calcium from the bones.

- The Gastrointestinal System:
Constipation and dry, difficult to evacuate stools are the result of immobility.

- The Psychological and Neurological Systems:
Some of the psychological hazards of immobility include lowered mood, frustration, and depression.

It is important that all clients are able to prevent further loss and ability. In order to ensure the client does not lose this, he/she is encouraged to stay as independent as possible and to achieve more independence when possible.

Rehabilitation and restorative care play a very important role in healthcare. People of all ages receive this special care in the hospital, nursing home, assisted living home, rehabilitation hospital, outpatient center, and even the person's own home.

When a patient receives rehabilitation and restorative care, he/she most often gets physical therapy, occupational therapy, and/or speech therapy, and the nursing assistant practices these learned skills with the patient. This care aims to restore lost ability and function and to prevent further loss of ability.

People of all ages receive rehabilitation and restorative care. Young children and infants may receive this care when they are born with a deformity, older children and teens may receive this care when they get a broken a limb from a sport such as football or snow skiing, and adults may receive this care after they have a serious operation or injury. Older adults are in the age group that most often receives rehabilitation and restorative care. This care is very often used for older patients who have had a stroke, hip fracture, cardiac disorder, or limb amputation or who have been on bed rest for a long time.

Older adults and younger people often have different treatment goals. The goal of care for an older person may be to help him/her be able to do one or more of the basic activities of daily living such as walking with a cane or walker. Other common goals for an older person are eating independently, getting in and out of the tub or shower, safely climbing up stairs, gripping items with a hand that has been weakened by a stroke, increasing strength and endurance, cooking meals using special cooking utensils (if needed), and communicating with others through the spoken word or a special word board.

Younger patients usually have different kinds of treatment goals because their physical problems are quite different from those of an older person. Rehabilitation and restorative care for the younger person most often aims to restore the person to full, normal function after an accident or injury. Some of these goals include returning to work and school; being able to perform usual routines and activities of daily living; having full mobility of a fractured joint, such as a knee, after surgery or a cast; and regaining body strength after a period of illness and/or hospitalization.

Rehabilitation and restorative care can be given to the patient in the hospital, in the nursing home, in an assisted living home, in a rehabilitation hospital, in an outpatient community rehabilitation center, and in the person's own home or apartment.

Most rehabilitation and restorative care is provided by physical therapists, occupational therapists, and speech therapists. Some hospitals, nursing homes, and rehabilitation centers also have physical therapy assistants, occupational therapy assistants, and rehabilitation and restorative aides who help with this care. These people are given special training and education so they can help the physical therapist, occupational therapist, and speech therapist in reaching the goals of care.

Physical therapists provide range of motion exercise, muscle strengthening, general conditioning exercises, coordination exercise, transfer training, and ambulation assistance.

Range of Motion Exercise

Physical therapists, nurses, and nursing assistants provide and encourage range of motion exercise to increase the patient's ability to move joints fully, especially after a long period of bed rest or immobility and/or a disorder that affects range of motion. Pain and lack of functional ability occur when a joint does not have normal range of motion.

Joints move in different ways. For example, some joints flex, such as bending at the elbow. Other joint movements include extension, such as straightening the arm at the elbow; hyperextension, such as bending the head forcibly backwards; abduction, which is movement of the bone toward the body; rotation, which is movement of the bone around its central axis; circumduction, which is movement of the distal part of the bone in a circle while the proximal end remains fixed; eversion, which is movement of the ankle joint when turning the sole of the foot outward; inversion, which is movement of the ankle joint when turning the sole of the foot inward; pronation, which is moving the forearms so the palms of the hands face down in front of the body; and supination, which is moving the forearms so the palms of the hands face upward in front of the body.

The three kinds of range of motion exercise are:

- Active Range of Motion:
  Active range of motion is used when the patient is able to perform full range of motion to one or more parts of his/her body without the physical help of another. Nursing assistants and other members of the healthcare team may simply have to remind the person to do these exercises and watch him/her to ensure that he/she is doing these exercises in the right way.

- Active-Assistive Range of Motion:
  Active-assistive range of motion is used when a patient needs some help performing full range of motion to one or more parts of the body because his/her muscles are too weak or stiff to perform these exercises on their own. The nursing

assistant and other members of the team must help this person with his/her range of motion.

- Passive Range of Motion:
  Passive range of motion is used for a patient who cannot move one or more parts of his/her body at all. For example, a patient in a coma needs passive range of motion to all joints. The nursing assistant and other members of the team will have to perform full range of motion for the patient without any help from him/her. This passive range of motion prevents deformity and loss of function.

At times, weights are used with active range of motion and active-assistive range of motion. Active-assistive and passive range of motion exercises are performed in a gentle, slow way so the joints and bones are not hurt or harmed. If the patient starts to feel pain, stop. These exercises are NOT performed to the point of pain, and they should NOT be performed on an area with an untreated fracture. Again, nursing assistants must document their range of motion exercises and report to the nurse any abnormal observations.

Muscle Strengthening Exercise

Muscle strengthening exercises are used for patients and residents of all ages. For an older person, the goal of these exercises may be to get strong enough to perform some basic activities of daily living such as combing his/her hair.

For a younger person, the goal of these exercises may be to restore weak muscles to full strength. For example, a baseball pitcher may need muscle strengthening exercises after an arm injury in order to return to the game.

General Conditioning Exercises

These exercises increase the function of the heart and lungs, maintain range of motion, and increase muscle strength.

Coordination Exercises

Coordination exercises are mostly used for enabling gross and fine motor functioning. Gross motor function includes activities such as walking; fine motor function includes the use of hands and fingers to manipulate things such as buttons and forks.

Transfer Training

Many people get rehabilitation and restorative care to enable them to move safely from the bed to the chair, from the bed or chair to the commode, and/or from a sitting to a standing position. The goal of this transfer training is to help the person move about in a safe way with the greatest amount of independence possible. Many people who have had a stroke or a bone fracture need transfer training.

Some people can bear weight on both legs; others cannot. When a person is unable to bear full and strong weight on both legs, he/she may need a cane, walker, chair with a high seat, and/or self-lifting chair for some transfers.

Ambulation Exercises

Ambulation exercises are frequently done as part of a patient's rehabilitation and restorative plan of care. A young person may need this form of exercise after surgery; an older person may need this form of exercise after a long illness and bed rest.

The purpose of these exercises is to help the patient walk safely without the help of another person. Some patients can be taught to ambulate independently with the help of a device such as a cane, crutches, a splint, a brace, or a walker; others may be able to walk without these assistive devices after ambulation exercises. Parallel bars and/or gait or ambulation belts are often used for these exercises and ambulation.

It is often necessary that the patient have range of motion, balance, and muscle strengthening and/or coordination exercises before ambulation exercises can be started.

Once the person is able to walk safely on a flat and level surface, he/she may then start walking up and down stairs using a handrail. When a person walks up the stairs, he/she should put up the good leg on the stair and then bring up the weak one.

Occupational therapists, like physical therapists, are also part of the rehabilitation and restorative care team. Some of the activities of daily living the occupational therapist helps with are dressing, grooming, mouth care, bathing and/or showering, feeding, cooking meals, and getting around in and caring for the home.

Some people need special assistive devices to perform activities of daily living. For example, a person may need special gripping devices to pick up items off the floor. Others may need special forks and eating utensils to better pick up food from their plate. Some may need special plates with high sides to keep food on the plate when a person has trouble with a spoon or fork. Others may need clothing made with large buttons or Velcro strips when they cannot handle small buttons and zippers.

Nursing assistants help patients and residents with activities of daily living, as planned by the occupational therapist and other members of the rehabilitation team. For example, nursing assistants should help patients dress and operate any special devices they use.

Speech therapists help patients with communication. They also help patients with a swallowing disorder, something that often occurs after a stroke. These therapists also use assistive devices. For example, they may use a word board so a patient who cannot speak can communicate his/her needs to others. For example, many older people after having a stroke and having their speech center damaged get speech therapy so they can speak. This lack of speech is often very upsetting to the patient.

Nursing assistants should encourage the patient or resident to speak whenever possible. When the person cannot speak, the nursing assistant and other team members should give him/her the communication tool given to the patient by the speech therapist. For example, if a person has a word board, encourage him/her to use it.

Devices Used for Rehabilitation and Restorative Care

Splints:
Splints are specially made items for a patient or resident to prevent a deformity, such as a contracture, and to promote function. Some examples of splints are hand splints, a wrist splint, and a foot drop splint.

Self-Help Devices:
Self-help devices help the patient or resident to function in a safe and independent way even though he/she has a disorder or physical problem.

Some examples of self-help devices are walkers; shower chairs; special combs and brushes for grooming; shoehorns for dressing without full range of motion; raised sitting chairs, raised toilet seats, and chair leg extenders for safe transfer without the help of another person; and cups with lids and special plates with deep centers and weight for eating meals without spilling.

Nursing assistants, patient-care technicians, physical therapy assistants, occupational therapy assistants, rehabilitation and restorative aides, nurses, and other members of the healthcare team support the work of the physical therapist, occupational therapist, and speech therapist by following the plan of care and working with the person in the nursing care unit so he/she can meet his/her rehabilitation and restorative goals.

Heat Therapy and Cold Therapy:
Heat increases the flow of blood to a body part, helps joint stiffness and pain, decreases muscle spasms, and halts swelling and inflammation.

Heat therapy is often used for short-term and chronic problems such as arthritis, strains, sprains, spasms, and neurological problems. It is applied with a heating pad or a moist heat pack. All heat must be administered very carefully. Heat can burn the patient's skin, especially when he/she does not feel heat because of poor nerve sensation and when he/she is mentally unable to communicate a burning feeling.

Sometimes cold is used immediately after an injury occurs. Cold decreases blood flow to the injured area and halts swelling after an injury has occurred.

Cold must also be given with care. It, too, can cause tissue damage (frost bite), and it can lower body temperature. Cold is administered with an ice bag or cold pack.

Ultrasound:

This treatment is done with sound waves. These sound waves travel deep into the body's tissues and produce heat. This form of therapy is used when the patient has a poor range of motion caused by shortened muscles, a disorder such as bursitis or tendonitis, and/or back pain.

Water Therapy:

Water therapy, also called hydrotherapy, uses moving water to apply heat to an area. Water therapy is used to help wound healing, relieve pain, and relax muscles. This therapy is often used along with range of motion exercises so that the muscles are relaxed and the patient can be pain-free while going through the range of motion.

Some water therapy is given using a Hubbard tank, which is a very large whirlpool bath. The water is usually heated to 96° to 104° F. Some patients and residents may feel weak and tired after water therapy, so safety must be maintained. At times, the patient's blood pressure may drop while in the whirlpool.

Electrical Nerve Stimulation:

Electrical nerve stimulation, using small electrodes, contracts muscles to keep them from going into a spasm, something that often happens when a person has hemiplegia as the result of a stroke or another disorder. It also prevents muscles from shrinking when they are not being used for one reason or another.

Some patients are given a transcutaneous electrical nerve stimulation (TENS) machine to use for back pain, arthritis, sprains, and other disorders.

Massage:

Massage is also done by physical therapists. Massage helps to reduce pain and swelling. It is used for patients and residents with a fracture, sprain, or strain or nerve injury. Many people with lower back pain, arthritis, bursitis, neuritis, hemiplegia, paraplegia, multiple sclerosis, and cerebral palsy are helped with massage.

SELF-CARE/INDEPENDENCE

As previously stated, patients should be encouraged to be as independent as possible in meeting personal and self-care needs. Aids that can be used to help the patient be more independent in the home and in the healthcare facility include:

- Graspers and reachers so the patient can easily and safely pick up items from the floor

- Button hooks and Velcro closures on clothing and shoes

- Zipper pulls for clothing

- Handwriting aids such as a triangular grip or cylindrical foam to position the fingers better and more comfortably to make writing easier and more legible

- Special eating utensils such as bowls, rocker knives, plates, and utensils

- Special jar openers

- Key holders that give the client adequate leverage to easily turn the key in the lock

- Bath mitts, shower chairs, step-in showers, grab bars, and back scrubbers

- Drawer knob and door knob devices specially adapted to the patient's needs

- A rising chair to enable the patient to rise from the chair

- Toileting aids such as raised toilet seats and bars surrounding the toilet

Chapter 4: Psychosocial Care Skills

EMOTIONAL AND MENTAL HEALTH NEEDS

Emotional and mental health needs are a large part of healthcare. All clients are different and therefore, require different emotional and mental healthcare. Some of the most commonly occurring psychological and emotional alterations associated will illnesses and disorders include anxiety, depression, grief and loss, alterations of bodily image, loss of control, coping, and coping skills.

Anxiety

Anxiety affects the client with feelings of dread, discomfort, and apprehension. Anxiety leads to autonomic responses and anticipation of danger.

The signs and symptoms of anxiety include:
- Increased helplessness, irritability, fright, and worry
- Insomnia and vigilance
- Anorexia, increased blood pressure, and increased pulse
- Diaphoresis and trembling
- Fatigue, urinary changes, weakness, and faintness
- Poor problem-solving skills and lack of an adequate attention span

Depression

Depression, of varying degrees, often affects the client and those close to the client when he/she is affected with a serious illness. Depression leads to physical, emotional, and cognitive changes.

The signs and symptoms of depression include:
- Feelings of poor self-esteem and worthlessness
- Sadness and despair
- Insomnia and sleep loss
- Listlessness
- Weight loss and anorexia
- Social withdrawal
- Lack of sexual desire
- Poor levels of concentration, poor decision-making and problem-solving skills, and diminished performance

At times, a depressed client is at risk for suicide. All threats of suicide must be taken seriously and must IMMEDIATELY be reported to the nurse.

The care and treatment for a depressed client is multifaceted. The client needs social and perhaps spiritual support; cognitive behavioral therapy; and often, medications such as antidepressants and non-pharmacological approaches such as stress reduction and relaxation techniques.

Delirium

Delirium is a serious disturbance to a patient's mental abilities. The primary symptoms of delirium are:

- Reduced awareness of the environment, an inability to stay focused on one topic, and being withdrawn

- Cognitive impairments such as disorientation; inability to recognize people, places, or things; rambling speech; poor short-term memory; fear, anxiety, depression, or anger; changes in sleep habits; restlessness; agitation; irritability; combative behavior; and hallucinations

Dementia

Alzheimer's syndrome is the number one cause of progressive dementia.

The signs and symptoms of dementia include hallucinations, delusions, memory loss, agitation, paranoia, personality changes, and problems performing usual activities. The client may have difficulty sleeping, may have problems with communication, and may also forget to take medications.

Grief and Loss

A loss can be actual, perceived, or anticipated. It occurs when a person undergoes a significant change that causes the loss of something valuable or when a person anticipates and/or perceives the loss of something valuable.

Sources of loss can originate from many things including from a loss of self and of one's bodily image, from the signs and symptoms of the disease or disorder, from extrapersonal losses such as the loss of a home in a fire, and from the loss of savings due to hospitalization and medical care. All losses impact the client.

Perceived losses are losses that are unverifiable by others. The client with a perceived loss experiences feelings of grief because he/she perceives a loss even though it is not actually occurring. For example, an elderly woman may perceive that she is no longer useful to others, when in fact the woman is still actively engaging in social and charitable activities. This perception, although faulty, still impacts and affects the person.

People have anticipatory grief and loss before an actual or perceived loss actually occurs. For example, a son may undergo severe anticipatory loss and grief soon after his mother has been diagnosed with a serious disease or disorder. Similarly, a woman may have anticipatory loss and grief relating to the loss of a limb that is infected as a result of her disease or disorder.

Patients coming to terms with diseases or disorders often experience a range of emotions including anger, fear, shock, disbelief, sadness, and depression.

SPIRITUAL AND CULTURAL NEEDS

Spiritual and Religious Needs

Although spirituality and religion are similar concepts, they are quite different. Religion has a formal set of practices, values, and beliefs that a person follows and practices in order to meet human challenges and to find the overall meaning and purpose of life. Spirituality is primarily informal and not based on a formal set of practices, values, and beliefs. Instead, spirituality is more personal and entails a desire to find meaning and to establish and maintain connectedness with others, the environment, and a higher being who is not necessarily God.

Spiritual and religious needs often increase with disease, illness, and injury. Some of these needs include the need for gratitude; the need to cope with loss; the need for meaning in terms of self; the need to be certain of, and believe in, a god or higher power; and the need to contribute to society and/or one's group.

Spiritual distress is a lack of spiritual well-being. Spiritual distress can be seen when the client verbalizes, or demonstrates non-verbally, that he/she has lost or fears losing a sense of purpose, hope, and/or meaning. This is also true when the patient feels abandoned or angry toward his/her god or higher power. Spiritual well-being occurs when the client has feelings about the meaning and purpose of life. Clients demonstrate and verbalize spiritual well-being when they express love, forgiveness, faith, and meaning of life.

Other concepts relating to religion and spirituality include forgiveness, faith, hope, and transcendence. Self-transcendence allows clients to reach out to things above and beyond them. They believe there is something greater than self.

The spiritual and religious beliefs, symbols, and practices that nursing assistants must be aware of include:

- Meatless Fridays during Lent for Roman Catholics and a Kosher diet for Jews
- Sacred writings including the Bible and the Koran
- Dress beliefs, which can include a Hindu saris and a Jewish Yamakah
- Beliefs relating to birth and death including the religious and spiritual belief of an afterlife and heaven
- Meditation and prayer
- Healing beliefs such as traditional religious healing ceremonies
- Sacred symbols such as the Christian cross, the Jewish star of David, and the Muslim mala

- Holy days, such as Christmas and Yom Kippur, and their meanings

Culture and Cultural Needs

Although the terms culture and ethnicity are sometimes used as synonyms, they are not. Culture is a set of practices, customs, beliefs, and attitudes passed on from generation to generation, which is not shared by others outside of the culture. An ethnic group shares a characteristic such as a language; race is based on a physical or genetic trait such as skin color. The U.S. is often referred to as a "melting pot" of many different cultures and people of virtually all ethnicities. Nursing assistants and other healthcare providers must accommodate each patient's specific cultural and ethnical needs in all aspects of care.

The culture of a client is important. Knowing the client's culture and cultural beliefs allows healthcare workers to better understand the client as a person. It greatly impacts the client's health and his/her reactions to treatments and care.

Cultures vary in opinions about family and the roles different members of the family serve. Different cultures have different beliefs regarding the size of the family and how family members communicate with each other. For example, some cultures believe the oldest members of the family are most important because they have lived the longest and therefore know the most. Other cultures focus on the father of the family as the decision-maker; others look at the mother as the decision-maker in the family.

Non-verbal and verbal communication varies among cultures. Some of the variations relating to verbal communication include the use of certain words, language, and speech qualities. Silence is also an example of a culturally varying pattern of communication. Some cultures accept it; others view it as a lack of interest from the healthcare provider.

Non-verbal communication patterns, other than silence, include touch, eye contact, gestures, body posture, and facial expressions. Touch, like silence, varies among cultures. Some cultures welcome and accept it; others consider it inappropriate, unacceptable, and invasive.

Facial expressions are interpreted by different people and different cultures in many different ways. Some cultures readily and frequently smile; others do not. Facial expressions are often difficult to interpret with certainty. For this reason, nursing assistants and other healthcare workers must explore all possible meanings of facial expressions and determine what the facial expressions are suggesting. For example, a client can look agitated and annoyed even though he/she simply is tired and in need of rest.

Eye contact, or lack thereof, also varies among cultures. Some cultures use and accept eye contact as a sign of honesty, interest, attentiveness, self-confidence, and good self-esteem. For these cultures, lack of eye contact can indicate guilt, lack of interest, inattentiveness, shyness, and even dishonesty. Other cultures consider eye contact invasive, aggressive, and rude.

Space and distance tolerance is also different among cultures. It appears that people who live in crowded areas are more tolerant of closeness than those accustomed to less crowded areas. American culture has four personal spaces:

- The *intimate zone* is from 6 inches to 1½ feet from the body. Most cultures view this space as highly personal and one that is guarded and protected from others unless the person has an intimate relationship with another person in this space. This space is often necessarily invaded by healthcare professionals when they provide care.

- The *personal space* is typically reserved for close, friendly interactions such as those common among family members and close friends. This space extends beyond the intimate zone, and it is from 1½ feet to 4 feet from the body.

- The *social zone* is tolerated when the client is interacting with strangers such as nursing assistants or other healthcare workers. It is defined as a distance of 4 feet to 12 feet from the body.

- The *public* zone is over 12 feet from the body. This space is typically used when a person is in a large crowd, such as occurs in group teaching.

Cultures also differ in terms of favorite foods, preferred methods of cooking, and the meaning of food. For example, Hispanic and Asian cultures prefer rice as a staple, and Indian people prefer unleavened bread. Foods are also associated with health among some cultures. "Hot" foods are used to treat "cold" diseases. For example, some cultures view corn meal as a "hot" food that can treat a "cold" disorder such as arthritis.

Food is also closely aligned with religious practices. For example, Roman Catholics do not eat meat on certain days such as Ash Wednesday and Good Friday; Orthodox Jews do not mix meats and dairy in the same meal; and Hindus, Sikhs, and Buddhists are vegetarians.

Chapter 5: Role of the Nurse Aide

The Role of the Nursing Assistant

Certified nursing assistants are a crucial part of a nursing program. The CNA is trained to safely bathe, groom, dress, and assist patients with activities of daily living. They are also trained to safely assist with ambulation, transfers, and bed mobility.

Additionally, the CNA training includes instructions on how to provide active and passive range of motion exercises. They are also educated to provide patients with basic massage, such as back rubs, and skin care to prevent breakdown. They also learn about nutrition and basic anatomy and physiology. The nursing aide may be called "the nurse" by many patients, but he/she works under the direction of a nurse and must adhere to the CNA scope of practice and report findings to the nurse.

COMMUNICATION

Communication is the act of conveying a message to another person through writing, speech, behaviors, and/or pictures. Communication is a dynamic, interactive, and highly active process during which messages are formed by the sender, transmitted by the sender, and received by the receiver.

The Components of the Communication Process

The *sender* transmits the message to others; the *receiver* is the person who gets the message from the sender. The sender and receiver alternate roles throughout a conversation as they respond and provide feedback to each other. The *channel* is the means with which the message is transmitted from the sender to the receiver. Examples of channels are vision and touch. The *message* is the feelings or information transmitted from the sender to the receiver.

A verbal or non-verbal response to a message sent from the receiver to the sender is called *feedback*. Feedback allows us to acknowledge that the message was received, to respond to the message, to seek clarification of the message, and/or to convey an understanding of the message. Feedback helps the sender to confirm that the message was accurately received and interpreted by the receiver.

Encoding and decoding occur when communication occurs between people. *Encoding* is the cognitive, or thinking, process the sender uses when considering how to frame or formulate the message. *Decoding* is the cognitive process the receiver uses to understand the message from the sender.

Factors That Impact the Communication Process

Factors that can positively and negatively impact communication include:
- Attitudes

- Culture
- Perceptions
- Differences in knowledge
- Past experiences
- Emotions
- Relationships and roles
- Environmental settings
- Physical discomfort
- Time pressures
- Language
- Values

Verbal Communication

Nursing assistants and patients simultaneously employ both verbal and non-verbal types of communication. Verbal communication, which is typically conscious, transmits messages through the written or spoken word.

Components of verbal communication include sounds, such as crying and groaning; the tone, pitch, and intonation of the sender's voice; the volume of speech; the rate or pace of the speech; the simplicity of the speech; the use of pauses; the clarity of the speech; the brevity of the discussion; the credibility of the sender; and the appropriate use of humor.

Sounds are often difficult to interpret accurately. Often, sounds can convey or express several emotions. Expressionless speech conveys to the client a lack of interest, and a loud voice and rapidly paced speech is often highly intimidating to the patient. Pauses can help the sender and receiver to consider the message and encode feedback; prolonged pauses can be awkward and uncomfortable for the client.

Short, clear, and simple messages are more easily understood by the patient, and these types of messages are less susceptible to misinterpretation.

Non-verbal Communication and Body Language

Non-verbal communication is far less conscious than verbal communication. Many consider non-verbal messages stronger and more powerful than words transmitted concurrently in a verbal message.

Some examples of non-verbal communication are:
- Gestures
- Touch
- Use of space
- Body movements or body language
- Facial expressions
- Eye movements
- Body posture and gait

- Personal appearance
- Congruency with the verbal message

Individuals communicate several feelings, emotions, and attitudes through their body movements, body language, and gestures. The way a person holds himself/herself, walks, stands, sits, and moves about can communicate negative feelings and emotions such as depression, fatigue, lack of interest, pain, and despair. Conversely, these factors can also communicate self-confidence, high self-concept, sense of well-being, and a positive and optimistic mood.

Eyes and eye movements are very revealing and reflective of a number of different things. Direct eye contact can convey openness, sincerity, a positive sense of self, and interest. Conversely, lack of eye contact can convey shyness, nervousness, embarrassment, dishonesty, defensiveness, and low self-esteem.

Touch, or tactile, communication conveys caring, compassion, and understanding; however, you must be aware that some individuals and cultures are not accepting of touch by members outside of the immediate family unit.

Facial expressions can transmit and convey happiness, sadness, surprise, impatience, disgust, fear, boredom, and anger, among a wide variety of other emotions. An emotionless face indicates a flat effect that may result from a lack of interest or some type of illness such as severe depression or Alzheimer's dementia, or it may be the patient's usual expression. Additionally, you must be constantly aware of patients' own facial expressions, other forms of non-verbal communication, and their effect on patients and family members.

Communicating with a patient at eye level, rather than from an upper position, makes the client more comfortable and able to openly communicate with the nursing assistant and other healthcare workers. This eye level positioning conveys equality, non-judgmental attitudes, and interest in the nursing assistant-client relationship.

Personal appearance strongly influences the initial impressions and perceptions people form about others. Criteria that provide this non-verbal data include manner of dress, style of hair, makeup, and degree of cleanliness.

Occasionally, the spoken word and the non-verbal message sent with facial expressions or other forms of non-verbal communication do not match; they are incongruent. It is then the nursing assistant's responsibility to clarify the meaning.

Written Communication

Written communication can include letters, notes, signs, cards, and emails. Medical records, which include doctor's notes, nurse's notes, and documentation from nursing assistants and other healthcare workers, are also a form of written communication.

Therapeutic Communication

The three requirements of therapeutic communication are respect, empathy, and positive sense of self.

Respect involves caring, warmth, interest, and no judgment about the patient or his/her feelings. You are responsible for accepting the person for who he/she is, not for what he/she thinks. This includes people with whom you may not agree.

Respecting a client includes calling him/her by name. If the patient is a child, call him/her by first name; if he/she is an adult, call him/her Mr. or Ms. plus the last name. Never, unless asked to, call an adult by his/her first name. Also never use terms of endearment such as honey, dear, sweetie, etc. as these do not show respect.

Do not refer to the client by his/her illness, surgery, or room number such as "the diabetic" or "room 64C." Clients are not room numbers and are not illnesses; they are people who should be treated with respect at all times.

Empathy refers to understanding the client's feelings, attitudes, values, and beliefs. You must respect that the client may have feelings dissimilar from yours. Listen carefully and attentively to what the client feels. Do not interject your feelings; the client has a right to feel however he/she wants.

Special Communication

It is important that nursing assistants and other healthcare personnel be able to communicate with clients in an effective manner. This means that both sending and receiving messages should be able to be performed. Clients must be able to understand all messages sent to them. Healthcare workers must also be able to understand all messages from clients.

Sending and receiving a message with a confused, sleepy, or unconscious person is never easy; it requires special skills. Special skills are also required when a person has a mental problem or illness. Use simple, plain words that a person can understand. Do not use words such as "NPO," "ambulate," or "void" if the person does not know their meaning. For example, say, "You can not eat or drink anything after 12 midnight" instead of saying "NPO." You may want to ask the person if he/she "would like to walk" instead of asking if he/she "would like to ambulate." Also, use the word "urinate" or show the male patient the urinal instead of using the word "void" unless he understands that word.

Other practices that can help the communication process include:

- Include the family and friends in the communication when a patient is unable to understand what you are trying to say.

- Ask the family and friends how the person can be helped to communicate with you.

- Talk to patients in a quiet place without many distractions. After asking the patient's permission, turn off the radio and television while talking to him/her.

- Ensure the person can see you; turn on the lights if the room is too dark.

- Keep the message as short and simple as possible. Many people do best with short talks rather than long ones with a lot of information given at one time. It is better to talk for a few short sessions instead of one or two long ones.

- Discuss one thing at a time.

- Repeat the message as often as needed.

- Ask one question at a time and listen to the answer.

- Draw pictures and let the client do the same.

- Ask "yes" or "no" questions.

- Speak slowly and clearly.

- Talk with a low-pitched voice, not a high-pitched one.

- Face the person to whom you are talking.

- Make eye contact with the person.

- Listen to the person.

- Look at the person's face. Is the patient trying to tell you something? Give the patient his/her eyeglasses and hearing aid if he/she wears them.

- Always show respect and caring.

- When a patient cannot understand the spoken word, communicate with touch and a calm voice when telling him/her you care.

CLIENT RIGHTS

In the U.S., all people have basic rights. All clients are awarded these basic rights as well as some additional ones. These additional rights are awarded to those in a hospital, assisted living home, and/or nursing home. When clients, whether outpatient or inpatient, seek or receive services from any of these places, they are given a copy of these rights so they can be sure they are treated properly.

Nursing assistants and all other healthcare workers must know these rights and ensure that any and all clients have them while being provided with care in the facility.

All clients have the right to the following:
- Accurate bills for services given
- Respect and dignity
- Their personal property
- To complain and be heard
- Confidentiality
- Privacy
- To know about his/her medical condition and treatments
- To choose his/her own doctors
- Competent care
- Religious and social freedom
- To make decisions about his/her medical care
- Freedom from abuse and neglect
- Control over his/her own money

Respect and Dignity

All people have a right to respect and dignity. This means that nursing assistants must:
- Address all clients and any other people by their names.
- Speak to clients and everyone else with respect in a kind, helpful, and respectful manner.
- Always treat and speak to others as you would like to be treated and spoken to.
- Make people feel special every time you speak to them or encounter them.
- Never treat an adult like a child. This includes never speaking to him/her in a childish or baby-like tone.
- Ensure all clients are kept clean and presentable at all times. Always use good communication skills. Ensure clients are awarded privacy, especially when they are bathing or changing clothes. Allow clients to express their thoughts and feelings whenever they choose.
- Allow clients to be as independent as possible. Always encourage independence and assist them, if necessary, with any activities of daily living.
- Always treat clients with dignity. Never allow them to stay wet with urine or dirty with a foul smell or odor.
- Give clients as many choices as possible.

Confidentiality

All clients have the right to keep their personal medical information confidential from everyone except those caring for them. It is the client's decision whether or not to tell others about his/her diagnosis and/or any other personal medical information.

There are confidentiality laws, called HIPAA laws, in place that protect client information. Nursing assistants and all other healthcare workers are responsible for honoring this confidentiality. In doing so, they must not discuss the client in areas where others may hear such as in hallways, the cafeteria, etc. This also includes not speaking about the client at home with family members or friends as well as ensuring that the client's files are kept in a safe and secure place where only care givers can access them.

Do not reveal any client's personal medical information over the phone. This is important, because you do not know who may be listening to the conversation. It must be the client's decision whether or not to share his/her information.

Privacy

Clients always have a right to privacy. Just because a client is in the hospital or other facility, it does not mean he/she has lost that right. This also remains true when a client receives home healthcare.

It is important to give the client privacy in any healthcare setting, even if care is provided in his/her home. When caring for a client, it is essential that his/her personal privacy is always protected. This includes when a client is changing or being changed, bathing or being bathed, when being examined, etc. Nursing assistants and all other healthcare personnel should always knock on the client's door before entering. The patient's room is his/her own private space, just as your room is to you.

Never open a client's closet or go into his/her pocketbook without permission. If you are providing care within the client's home, never enter any part of the house or open any closets, cabinets, or drawers without permission. Give the client privacy when he/she converses with family, friends, and any other clients or visitors including doctors. If the client needs a quiet and private place to hold a conversation, accommodate him/her.

The Right to Competent Care

Safe and high-quality care is another right of all clients. This includes the care from nursing assistants, nurses, doctors, and all other healthcare personnel. In order for the client to receive this type of care, all healthcare workers caring for him/her must know how to do so correctly.

If ever faced with a situation in which you are unsure what to do or how to do it, stop immediately and consult the nurse for instructions or explanations. Never under any circumstances do anything of which you are not 100% sure.

Religious and Social Freedom

Everyone in the U.S. has the right to religious and social freedom. Clients in the hospital or any other healthcare facility also have this freedom. Nursing assistants must respect this right for all clients.

Nursing assistants should:

- Never force any clients to attend any religious activity they do not wish to attend
- Always help clients attend the religious activities they choose to attend
- Encourage clients to choose whatever groups and activities they wish
- Help clients attend any social, recreational, and/or other activities they wish to attend, even if nursing assistants do not believe in those activities

Freedom from Abuse and Neglect

All humans should be free from abuse and neglect. Many elders, children, and young adults with physical or mental problems are at risk for abuse and neglect. Family members, care givers, healthcare workers, and other members of a community can abuse or neglect others.

Abuse is defined as maltreatment. Anyone can be abused: men, women, adults, children, and people of all ages. Child abuse is the maltreatment of infants and young children. Parents, relatives, and daycare providers are sometimes guilty of child abuse. Elder abuse affects older adults. The elderly person is usually abused by someone he/she trusts such as a son, daughter, spouse, nurse, nursing assistant, or home health aide. Elder abuse can occur in the home, assisted living facility, group home, or long-term care nursing home.

Nursing assistants and other healthcare workers must, by law in many states, immediately report all cases of suspected elder abuse and child abuse. When you suspect someone is abusing or neglecting a patient or resident, report it immediately. You do not need to be completely sure of the abuse in order to report it.

The different types of abuse are:

- Physical Abuse:
  Physical abuse is the use of a physical force such as a punch, slap, push, or pinch. Grabbing a person out of his/her bed is physical abuse. Signs of physical abuse include skin tears, bruises, and broken bones.

- Sexual Abuse:
  Sexual abuse is sexual contact of any kind without the consent of the other person. Touching, fondling, and rape are examples of sexual abuse.

- Financial Abuse:
  Financial abuse is the improper or illegal use of a person's money. Taking money from an elder to use for something he/she does not want is an example of financial abuse.

Neglect is a bit different than abuse. Neglect does not involve a wrongful act. Neglect is not doing something that should be done. Men, women, and people of all ages can be neglected.

The different types of neglect are:

- Physical Neglect:
  Not giving a person food or physical care he/she needs is an example of physical neglect.

- Emotional Neglect:
  Ignoring a person and abandoning a person who is afraid of being alone are examples of emotional neglect.

- Financial Neglect:
  An elder living with his/her daughter who does not let the elder buy eyeglasses with his/her own money is an example of financial neglect.

LEGAL AND ETHICAL BEHAVIOR

Legal and ethical behavior is essential to the nursing assistant and all other members of the healthcare team.

Legal Issues

Nursing assistants are responsible for knowing about legal behavior including:
- Scope of practice
- Standards of care
- Abandonment
- Negligence
- Criminal negligence
- Malpractice

Scope of Practice:
The scope of practice for nursing assistants and all other healthcare professionals is dictated by the individual states. These scopes of practice indicate what each profession can and cannot do. For example, the scope of practice for a registered nurse may allow him/her to dispense all medications, whereas the scope of practice for a nursing assistant may allow him/her to assist a client with self-care activities and to take vital signs.

Nursing assistants cannot do anything outside their scope of practice, or they risk violating the law. You must be familiar with your state's scope of practice for nursing assistants and refuse to do anything not included in it.

Standards of Care:
Standards of care are acceptable levels of care. For example, a standard of care can state what a nursing assistant must do if he/she sees a patient fall such as calling for help, staying with the fallen person, and/or examining the person for signs of harm from the fall. By not performing these actions, you would not be following the standards of care.

Nursing assistants can be held responsible for any harm or damage done to a client if they do not do what is expected of them. Standards of care are developed in healthcare policies and procedures, by organization and associations, and by the state.

Abandonment:
Abandonment is when a nursing assistant or other healthcare worker leaves a client without providing needed care. For example, if a nursing assistant is working an 11 p.m. to 7 a.m. shift and leaves early without informing the nurse, he/she has abandoned patients.

Negligence:
When a nursing assistant does not act the way he/she is supposed to, it is considered negligence. For instance, if a nursing assistant does not help a client eat dinner and take a bath, the nursing assistant is being negligent.

Criminal Negligence:
When a healthcare worker is very reckless with a client, he/she is being criminally negligent. For example, if a nursing assistant leaves a client who is at risk for falls in the bathtub unattended for an extended period of time and he/she falls and dies, the nursing assistant is considered to be criminally negligent.

Malpractice:
It is considered malpractice when a healthcare worker does not provide to a client the same level of care that he/she was taught in school, which leads to client injury or damage. An example is when a nursing assistant disregards the hand washing policy, which leads to a patient getting a serious infection. The nursing assistant can be guilty of malpractice because he/she was taught to wash the hands before and after all patients.

Unprofessional Conduct:
Unprofessional conduct is when a nursing assistant or any other healthcare worker does not follow the standards of practice, even if no harm or injury results from it. For example, it is considered unprofessional conduct for a nursing assistant to work under the influence of drugs or alcohol, even if no patients are harmed and no negative effects result from it.

Assault and Battery:
Assault occurs when someone fears that he/she will be touched, injured, or hurt without his/her permission. Telling someone that you will punch him/her if he/she does not shut up is an example of assault.

Battery is the actual touching, injuring, or hurting that occurs without a person's permission. If a nursing assistant or any other healthcare worker slaps, pushes, or causes any intentional harm to a client, it is considered battery. Battery also occurs when a nursing assistant forces a patient to eat or get a treatment after he/she has refused it.

Confidentiality:
As discussed above, breaking confidentiality is a violation of the HIPAA law.

Ethical Issues

The ethical principles that nursing assistants must abide by during all aspects of nursing care and practice include:

- Justice:
  The principle of justice requires nursing assistants to be fair to all. For example, limited resources, such as time and supplies, must be fairly and justly distributed among patients. All patients should be treated equally.

- Fidelity:
  Fidelity is being faithful to one's promises. The very nature of the nursing assistant-patient relationship requires that nursing assistants be faithful and true to his/her professional promises and responsibilities by providing safe, high-quality care in a competent manner while upholding client choices, desires, and innate rights.

- Beneficence:
  Although beneficence may appear to be the opposite of non-maleficence, it is not. Simply stated, beneficence means "do good." Doing good is more than just not doing harm.

- Non-maleficence:
  Non-maleficence means "do not harm," as stated in the Hippocratic Oath. Harm can be intentional or unintentional. When a client has an adverse effect, such as respiratory arrest resulting from a drug, it is considered unintentional harm. If, however, a nursing assistant pushes a patient to the floor, it is considered intentional harm and is a serious violation of law and ethics.

- Accountability:
  All nursing assistants are responsible for and accountable for all aspects of nursing care. They must answer to themselves, their clients, and society at large for their actions. They must also accept any and all personal and professional consequences for their actions.

- Autonomy and Self-Determination:
  Each unique individual has the right to make choices without coercion and the undue influence of others. Nursing assistants must never impose their own beliefs, values, or opinions on the client. They accept all client choices without judgment. The patient has the right to choose and/or refuse any and all treatments and interventions.

- Veracity:
  Veracity is truthfulness. Nursing assistants must always tell the entire truth and be truthful and honest with patients.

The number of ethical dilemmas and conflicts are rising because of several factors, including the wide variety and diversity of treatment options and the ongoing debate about who should receive limited resources. Many healthcare facilities have multidisciplinary ethics committees that resolve ethical dilemmas and conflicts.

MEMBERS OF THE HEALTHCARE TEAM

There are a wide variety of healthcare team members, including medical staff, nursing staff, rehabilitation/restorative staff, diagnostic staff, dietary staff, and respiratory staff.

Medical Staff

Some medical doctors work as part of a hospital staff for a medical specialty, primary care, or a specialty area such as the emergency department or critical care area. Others work in the community, but have privileges to practice in a particular healthcare facility. Many have specialty areas of practice such as geriatrics, obstetrics, or oncology; others are generalists who practice internal medicine or primary care.

Other medical roles include doctors of osteopathy (DO), doctors of optometry (OD), and doctors of chiropractic medicine. Additionally, medical physician extenders, such as physician assistants and nurse practitioners, perform limited roles in all types of healthcare settings and in all levels of care.

Nursing Staff

Members of the nursing team typically include registered nurses, licensed practical (or vocational) nurses, nursing assistants, and clerical help. Additional nursing staff in some facilities can also include patient-care technicians, nursing technicians, and telemetry aides, among other roles.

The registered nurse assesses, plans, implements, and evaluates client care; he/she also supervises staff, delegates assignments, provides patient education, and performs a number of other functions. The licensed practical nurse assists the registered nurse by collecting assessment data and providing direct care to patients that includes medication administration, sterile treatments such as wound care, and other tasks under the direction and supervision of the registered nurse.

Nursing assistants, patient-care technicians, nursing technicians, and similar workers are referred to as unlicensed assistive personnel. Although they may be "certified" by the state or healthcare facility, they are not licensed. These assistive staff members provide care to individual patients and groups of patients primarily in the areas of activities of daily living, mobility, nutrition, and hydration. They do NOT do anything that requires sterilization, and they are also supervised by the registered nurse.

Rehabilitation/Restorative Staff: Physical, Occupational, and Speech Therapists

Physical therapists assess, plan, implement, and evaluate interventions, including those related to strength, mobility, balance, gait, coordination, and range of motion. At times, the physical therapist may have the assistance of physical therapy assistants or physical therapy aides.

Occupational therapists assess, plan, implement, and evaluate interventions, including those that help clients to achieve the highest possible level of independence in terms of activities of daily living. Occupational therapists assess the need for and provide the client with adaptive devices such as special cutlery to facilitate independent eating and special devices to manipulate buttoning so the client can dress independently.

Speech pathologists/therapists assess, diagnose, and treat any communication and swallowing disorders. For example, a speech therapist may help the client form words when he/she is affected with expressive aphasia, may employ assistive devices such as word boards, and may actively collaborate with a dietitian in terms of nutrition for a client with a swallowing disorder that can lead to aspiratory and respiratory compromise.

Diagnostic Staff

Healthcare facilities have a number of diagnostic departments and staff that often collaborate with the nursing assistant. For example, the nursing assistant may collect and transport a specimen to the laboratory for testing; the nursing assistant may also transport a client to the radiology department for an X-ray, CT scan, or MRI. All of these areas have diagnostic staff.

Phlebotomist

Phlebotomists collect blood for donation or analysis in a clinical laboratory. Blood tests are used to diagnose illness, evaluate the effectiveness of medications, and determine whether or not a patient is receiving proper nutrition.

Laboratory Technician

A laboratory technician, also referred to as a clinical laboratory technician, is a person who, under the supervision of a medical technologist or physician, performs microscopic and bacteriologic tests of human blood, tissue, and fluids for diagnostic and research purposes.

Radiology Technician

A radiology technician, also referred to as a radiologic technologist or radiographer, is a medical worker who specializes in the production of medical images. This is not the same as a radiologist who is a medical doctor who specializes in interpreting these images.

Dietary Staff

Dietitians develop and oversee nutritional programs for several types of institutions, including schools, hospitals, and nursing homes.

Dietary aides perform important roles in hospitals, nursing homes, schools, and other institutions. Individuals looking for a job in which they can help other people should consider working as a dietary aide.

Respiratory Therapists

Respiratory therapists perform a number of different tasks, including collaborative patient assessment and planning as well as diagnostic procedures such as drawing arterial blood gas specimens. They also are responsible for provision of care, including managing respiratory treatments such as nebulizers, CPAP, and BPAP; setting up and maintaining mechanical ventilation; assisting the client with respiratory exercises; and administering respiratory-related medications and drugs.

Test Your Knowledge

1. Rehabilitation programs are:
    A. Specialized for each individual client
    B. The same for all clients
    C. The same for all stroke clients
    D. The same for all children

2. Select the nursing system that is correctly paired with its description.
    A. Supportive-educative nursing system: Meets the self-care needs of clients who can perform some, but not all, self-care functions.
    B. Wholly compensatory nursing system: Provides all care to the client because he/she is not able to perform any self-care.
    C. Wholly compensatory nursing system: Meets the self-care needs of clients who can perform some, but not all, activities of daily living.
    D. Partly compensatory nursing system: Provides all care to the client because he/she is not able to perform any self-care.

3. When bathing a client, the nursing assistant should check the:
    A. Condition of the skin
    B. Balance and gait
    C. Goss motor function
    D. Fine motor coordination

4. All clients should be bathed:
    A. In the morning
    B. In the middle of the day
    C. In the evening
    D. When they choose

5. Select the precaution that is correctly paired with its description.
    A. Standard precautions: Prevent any direct and indirect droplet transmissions, as can occur with diarrhea, wounds, and skin infections.
    B. Contact precautions: Apply to all blood and bodily fluids and all clients regardless of the person's diagnosis.
    C. Airborne precautions: Require the use of a special mask, called a HEPA mask, and a special negative pressure room.
    D. Droplet precautions: Apply to all blood and bodily fluids and all clients regardless of the person's diagnosis.

6. When giving a client a sponge bath, the height of the bed should be:
    A. As low as possible
    B. As high as possible
    C. Set in the middle
    D. Set at a comfortable working height

7. The water temperature for showering should be no:
    A. More than 95° F
    B. Less than 95° F
    C. Less than 110° F
    D. More than 110° F

8. What type of toothbrush is recommended for clients?
    A. Hard toothbrushes
    B. Soft toothbrushes
    C. Medium toothbrushes
    D. Medium to hard toothbrushes

9. If you put on gloves and then go to your client's room, you can:
    A. Wear the gloves to empty the client's bedpan
    B. Wear the gloves to change linens and clean the bathroom
    C. Wear the gloves to feed the client
    D. Not do any of the above

10. HEPA stands for:
    A. Health-effective particle avoidance
    B. Healthy efficient particle avoidance
    C. High-efficiency particulate absorption
    D. Highly efficient particulate absorbers

11. Oral hygiene should be performed:
    A. In the morning and evening only
    B. Several times a day, including morning, evening, before sleep, and before and after eating
    C. In the morning, evening, and before bed
    D. Before each meal

12. Dentures should be cared for:
    A. After mouth care
    B. Before and after mouth care
    C. Before mouth care
    D. Only if the client wants them to be cared for

13. If a client is unable to take a shower or bath, his/her hair:
    A. Can be washed with dry shampoo or with the help of a bed tray
    B. Cannot be washed
    C. Can be washed only once a week
    D. Can be washed only every other day

14. A warning sign of a pressure ulcer is:
    A. When pink skin on a bony area turns white
    B. When white skin on a bony area turns pink
    C. When white skin on a fatty area turns red
    D. A client who moves a lot during the day and night

15. Toenails should never be cut on:
    A. Any clients
    B. On any male clients
    C. On any female clients
    D. On clients with diabetes

16. The body is made up mostly of:
    A. Blood
    B. Water
    C. Muscles
    D. Tendons

17. What is the name for the state of a client who does not have enough fluids?
    A. Cardiac arrest
    B. Hormone-resistant
    C. Water-retained
    D. Dehydrated

18. If a room fills with smoke, everyone must:
    A. Run to the stairs
    B. Get low and go
    C. Open all doors and windows
    D. Stop and stand up

19. Fiber helps to prevent:
    A. Constipation
    B. Urinary incontinence
    C. Heart attacks
    D. Lung cancer

20. Infection control measures are used to prevent:
    A. Clients from switching beds
    B. Fevers and dehydration
    C. Fluid overloads and deficits
    D. Spread of germs

21. Germs are:
    A. The size of a checker
    B. Larger than a pea
    C. Small and invisible
    D. About 10mm long and 12mm wide

22. Germs are able to leave the body:
    A. Only through intimate contact
    B. During eating
    C. Through bowel movements
    D. Only during surgery

23. The most effective way that nursing assistants and other healthcare workers can avoid spreading germs and infections from clients to themselves and/or others is through proper:
    A. Feeding of clients
    B. Hand washing
    C. Bathing of clients
    D. Nail care of clients

24. Proper hand washing should take about:
    A. 20 seconds
    B. 10 seconds
    C. 8 minutes
    D. 5 minutes

25. Sitting on a patient's bed is:
    A. Permitted with the patient's permission
    B. Allowed only when tending to hygiene needs
    C. Never allowed
    D. Allowed only while helping the patient dress

26. What color indicates biohazards?
    A. Red
    B. Black
    C. Clear
    D. Green

27. If a client has an airborne contagious disease, which type of mask may be required?
    A. HIPPA
    B. HESA
    C. HIPAA
    D. HEPA

28. MRSA stands for:
    A. Methicillin-Resistant Synonymous Aureas
    B. Methicillin-Resistant Staphylococcus Aureus
    C. Morning Resource Syndrome Atrophy
    D. Methicillin Resource Syndrome Atrophy

29. If a client's clothes are on fire, you should:
    A. Try to pat down the fire with your hands
    B. Turn the fan in the room on high
    C. Tell the client to stop, not run
    D. Run and don't stop

30. If a nursing assistant forgets to document the client's urine output at the end of his/her shift, this is a mistake of:
    A. Omission
    B. Commission
    C. Remission
    D. Admission

31. If a nursing assistant brings the wrong client to the operating room for surgery, this is a mistake of:
    A. Admission
    B. Remission
    C. Commission
    D. Omission

32. Healthcare facilities view mistakes as an opportunity to:
    A. Find out which employee committed them
    B. Reprimand the employee who committed the mistakes
    C. Fix the mistakes and change the documentation
    D. Fix the procedures and processes that failed

33. The nursing assistant must report to the nurse:
    A. Every time something is unusual or abnormal
    B. Whenever the nurse is not too busy
    C. At the end of his/her shift
    D. Only if the nurse asks you to report

34. Identification should be performed:
    A. Every time the nursing assistant enters the client's room
    B. On clients whom the nursing assistant is not familiar
    C. Only when clients are admitted or released
    D. Only on clients who tend to wander off

35. Which clients should be screened for falls?
    A. The elderly
    B. The elderly and confused
    C. The elderly, the confused, and the mentally ill
    D. All clients

36. If a client must be transported by wheelchair and the only available wheelchair has a broken lock, what should the nursing assistant do?
    A. Use his/her foot to act as a lock on the wheelchair that is not working
    B. Transfer the client to a flat area where the locks are not necessary
    C. Don't use the wheelchair; report it and wait for another available wheelchair
    D. Allow the client to use a walker, and assist him/her carefully

37. The emergency room is very busy, and you are asked to apply restraints to a combative patient. You are unsure how to do this. What should you do?
    A. Apply the restraints and make sure the client is in a locked room away from everyone else
    B. Apply the restraints and stay in the room with the client until he/she calms down
    C. Explain to the nurse that you are unsure of how to apply the restraint
    D. Ask the client's loved ones to assist you in restraining him/her

38. When a client wanders off, it is referred to as:
    A. Elopement
    B. Delopement
    C. An escape
    D. Sundowning

39. What should you do if a client asks for a glass of water at 2 a.m.?
    A. Get a glass of water with a spill-proof top
    B. Check to make sure he/she is not NPO after midnight
    C. Ask the client if he/she wants cold or room temperature water
    D. Get the water and assist him/her as necessary

40. Select the type of fire extinguisher with its correct description.
    A. A: Can put out electrical fires
    B. B: Can put out fires on liquids and gases, but not electrical
    C. C: Can put out fires on paper, wood, and cloth, but not grease or electrical
    D. AB: Can put out electrical, liquid, and gas fires

41. What three things are necessary for a fire to start?
    A. A flammable liquid, solid, and gas
    B. A match, an area to burn, and carbon dioxide
    C. Carbon dioxide, a flame, and something to burn
    D. Heat, air, and something to burn

42. What does R-A-C-E stand for?
    A. React, Alert, Contain or Confine, Exit
    B. React, Alert, Contain or Confine, Extinguish
    C. Rescue, Alarm, Contain or Confine, Extinguish
    D. Rescue, Alert, Contain or Confine, Exit

43. What is the first step in managing stress?
    A. Identifying the source of the stress
    B. Determining how to get rid of the stress
    C. Breathing exercises
    D. Viewing the situation differently

44. The P-A-S-S method is used for:
    A. Checking a client's blood pressure
    B. Performing CPR on children
    C. Performing CPR on infants
    D. Operating a fire extinguisher

45. The root cause analysis team looks at:
    A. Urine output levels
    B. Nursing assistant interactions
    C. Nursing assistant performance ratings
    D. Errors and/or mistakes

46. Vital signs include the assessment of:
    A. Body temperature, pulses, blood tests, and blood pressure
    B. Body temperature, pulses, respirations, and blood pressure
    C. Body temperature, blood tests, respirations, and blood pressure
    D. Body temperature, blood tests, pulses, and blood pressure

47. The higher of the two blood pressure numbers is called:
    A. Systematic
    B. Systolic
    C. Diastolic
    D. Dysrhythmia

48. In which location can a pulse be taken?
    A. The chin
    B. The right side of the back
    C. The groin area
    D. The lower back on the left side

49. The carotid artery is located near the:
    A. Forehead
    B. Underarm
    C. Wrist
    D. Neck

50. Where is the femoral pulse located?
    A. The neck
    B. The groin area
    C. The forearm
    D. The wrist

51. Respiration rates are counted:
    A. From exhale to inhale
    B. From inhale to next inhale
    C. From inhale to exhale
    D. From inhale to heart beat

52. The first part of cardiopulmonary resuscitation (CPR) is:
    A. Mouth-to-mouth breathing
    B. Chest compressions
    C. Oxygen face mask
    D. One compression followed by one breath

53. Which part(s) of the body are the most important to keep oxygen flowing into when performing CPR?
    A. The brain
    B. The lungs and brain
    C. The heart and lungs
    D. The heart and brain

54. What does C-A-B of CPR stand for?
    A. Circulation Airway Breathing
    B. Circulating Airway Breaths
    C. Circulating Air to Breathe
    D. Circulation of Airborne Breaths

55. When a 6-year-old child needs CPR and no one else is around, what should be done first?
    A. Call 911 for help
    B. Perform CPR for 2 minutes before calling 911
    C. Perform CPR for 3 minutes before calling 911
    D. Perform CPR for 4 minutes before calling 911

56. When performing CPR on a 13-year-old, chest compressions should be:
    A. Four to six inches deep
    B. Performed only after signed parental consent
    C. Performed with two hands
    D. Performed with one hand

57. Which of the following CPR actions is used for a 6-year-old boy?
    A. Four to six-inch deep compressions
    B. Ten compressions to five breaths
    C. Compressions with one hand
    D. Compressions with two hands

58. Select the correctly paired age and CPR statement.
    A. Infant: Cover the entire mouth and nose with your mouth
    B. Infant: Use only one hand for compressions
    C. 4-year-old: Use two hands for compressions
    D. Adult: Chest compressions at a rate of 50 compressions per minute

59. How deep are adult compressions?
    A. 4-6 inches
    B. 4 inches
    C. 3 inches
    D. 2 inches

60. When administering CPR to an 18-year-old, how many compressions per breaths should be given?
    A. 20 compressions to 2 breaths
    B. 30 compressions to 2 breaths
    C. 40 compressions to 4 breaths
    D. 50 compressions to 4 breaths

61. When caring for a conscious person who is choking, in what position should your hands be?
    A. One hand in a fist under the rib cage and the other on the client's shoulder
    B. Both hands in fists on the lower abdomen
    C. Both hands open and pressing on the lower to mid abdomen
    D. One hand in a fist and the other grabbing the wrist of the fisted hand

62. Angela, a nursing assistant, bathes three clients. When is the proper time to document this?
    A. At the end of her shift
    B. After each bath is given
    C. After all the baths are given
    D. When she is finished with her dinner break

63. If a nursing assistant observes an abnormal-colored area on her client's leg, she should:
    A. Apply cream to the colored area
    B. Ask the client if he/she would like some cream to put on the spot
    C. Document it and report it to the nurse
    D. Ask the client if it itches; if it does, offer him/her anti-itch cream

64. How long should you rest a client's heart before taking his/her blood pressure?
    A. 5 minutes
    B. 10 minutes
    C. 15 minutes
    D. 20 minutes

65. A rocker knife is an example of a:
    A. Tool used for surgery
    B. Tool used to help open medication bottles
    C. Device that can help a client cut food.
    D. Device that moves clients in bed

66. Which type(s) of losses impact clients?
    A. Losses they see
    B. Losses they hear about
    C. All types of losses
    D. Losses they think may occur

67. What is the kind of grief or loss that occurs before an actual or perceived loss actually occurs?
    A. Perceived
    B. Actual
    C. Participatory
    D. Anticipatory

68. The Theory of Transcultural Nursing is also referred to as:
    A. The Caring Theory
    B. The Culture Care Diversity and Universality Theory
    C. The Universe Theory
    D. The Caring and Universal Theory

69. Which of the following is an example of non-verbal communication?
    A. Eye contact
    B. Whispering
    C. Intonation
    D. Yelling

70. Select the zone that is correctly matched with its distance from the body.
    A. The intimate zone: 6 inches to 1 ½ feet
    B. The personal zone: over 4 feet to 12 feet
    C. The social zone: over 12 feet
    D. The public zone: 1 ½ feet to 4 feet

71. Delirium usually comes on or appears:
    A. Within 3-6 months
    B. Very slowly
    C. Very quickly
    D. Sometimes slowly and sometimes quickly

72. Which of the following is an example of a lack of spiritual well-being?
    A. A lack of religion
    B. A lack of religious practices
    C. Spiritual affinity
    D. Spiritual distress

73. Which of the following is simply defined as the spiritual belief that all people make mistakes as a function of human nature?
    A. Transcendence
    B. Hope
    C. Forgiveness
    D. Faith

74. Select the position that is correctly matched with its pressure points.
    A. Semi-Fowlers Position: Male genitals, breasts, shoulder, cheek, and ears
    B. Lateral or Side Lying Position: Toes, knees, male genitals, breasts, shoulder, cheek, and ears
    C. Fowler's Position: Elbows, scapulae, and back of the head
    D. Supine or Back Lying Position: Toes, knees, male genitals, breasts, shoulder, cheek, and ears

75. In order to avoid choking, the client must be upright after eating for at least:
    A. 15 minutes
    B. 20 minutes
    C. 25 minutes
    D. 30 minutes

76. Which of the following is an example of mental neglect?
    A. Leaving a client alone when you know he/she this is fears being alone
    B. Refusing a client the food necessary to thrive
    C. Refusing a client eyeglasses when there are ample funds to buy them
    D. Refusing a client request for help when you can help him/her

77. If a nursing assistant administers narcotic medication to a client, he/she is:
    A. Operating within his/her scope of practice
    B. Operating outside his/her scope of practice
    C. Legally helping the nurse
    D. Legally helping the physician

78. When a nursing assistant or other healthcare worker leaves a client without providing him/her with needed care, it is considered:
    A. Standards of care
    B. Malpractice
    C. Neglect
    D. Assault and battery

79. Which of the following is an example of physical elder abuse?
    A. Treating an elder like a child
    B. Locking an elder in a room
    C. Punching an elder
    D. Threatening an elder

80. Which is an example of joint extension?
    A. Bending the elbow
    B. Moving the forearm
    C. Bending the head forward
    D. Straightening the arm at the elbow

81. What are the three critical elements of therapeutic communication?
    A. Respect, empathy, and positive sense of self
    B. Respect, emotion, and position for one's self
    C. Respect, emotion, and positive sense of self
    D. Respect, empathy, and position for one's self

82. A new client, whose full name is John M. Willard, should be called by the nursing assistant as:
    A. John Willard
    B. Mr. Willard
    C. John
    D. Willard

83. When a nursing assistant wants to discuss John M. Willard, a diabetic client in room 6, how should the nursing assistant refer to him?
    A. John, the diabetic in 6
    B. The diabetic patient in 6
    C. Mr. Willard
    D. The diabetic client in room 6

84. Which of the following is an example of an open-ended question?
    A. How was your day?
    B. Tell me what you did today.
    C. Did you like what you had for lunch?
    D. Were you given a bath today?

85. Which of the following is an example of a closed-ended question?
    A. Are you tired?
    B. Tell me what you liked about your dinner.
    C. What types of activities are you interested in?
    D. What kinds of fruits and vegetables do you like to eat?

86. Which of the following is NOT an example of a communication stopper?
    A. Probing
    B. Poor body language
    C. Rejection
    D. Open-ended question

87. Which of the following is an example of hyperextension?
    A. Movement of the ankle joint when turning the sole of the foot inward
    B. Movement of the bone around its central axis
    C. Movement of the bone toward the body
    D. Forceful backward movement of the head

88. The client's bills should reflect:
    A. Anything for which the client's insurance company agrees to pay
    B. All services a client is offered, even those he/she does not receive
    C. Services and items the client actually received
    D. Only the services for which the insurance company will pay full price

89. Which of the following is an example of speaking to a client with respect and dignity?
    A. "I'm sorry, Mr. Gregory. I do not have any extra pillows with me, but I will get one for you."
    B. "Ok, dear, I will be sure to get the nurse for you right away."
    C. "Of course, sweetheart. I will be happy to do that for you."
    D. "Yes, honey, it is almost time for dinner."

90. Who is legally allowed to look at a client's medical records?
    A. The client's wife
    B. The doctor caring for the client
    C. The client's visitors
    D. The client's immediate family

91. If a client asks a question and you are not 100 % sure of the answer, you should:
    A. Ignore him/her
    B. Take a guess
    C. Tell the client you are unsure and follow up with the nurse for the correct answer
    D. Tell the client the answer you are most sure is correct

92. A nursing assistant going to work under the influence of drugs or alcohol is an example of:
    A. Assault
    B. Battery
    C. Criminal malpractice
    D. Unprofessional conduct

93. What should a nursing assistant do if asked to do something outside his/her scope of practice?
    A. Document it
    B. Do it before documenting it
    C. Do it after documenting it
    D. Consult the nurse

94. Which member of the healthcare team assesses the client and works with the client to help make informed choices in regards to the nursing process?
    A. Physical therapist
    B. Occupational therapist
    C. Nurse
    D. Pharmacist

95. Which member of the healthcare team assesses, plans, implements, and evaluates interventions related to strength, mobility, balance, gait, coordination, and range of motion?
    A. Physical therapist
    B. Speech therapist
    C. Occupational therapist
    D. Nursing assistant

96. Which member of the healthcare team assesses, plans, implements, and evaluates interventions, including those that help clients achieve the highest possible level of independence in terms of activities of daily living?
    A. Occupational therapist
    B. Physical therapist
    C. Nursing assistant
    D. Speech therapist

97. Which member of the healthcare team assesses, diagnoses, and treats any communication and/or swallowing disorders?
    A. Occupational therapist
    B. Speech therapist
    C. Nursing assistant
    D. Physical therapist

98. Which member of the healthcare team draws arterial blood gas specimens?
    A. Nursing assistant
    B. Psychiatrist
    C. Occupational therapist
    D. Respiratory therapist

99. Which type of doctor is an OD?
    A. Doctor of osteopathy
    B. Doctor of orthopedics
    C. Doctor of optometry
    D. Doctor of ophthalmology

100. Which type of doctor is a DO?
    A. Doctor of optometry
    B. Doctor of osteopathy
    C. Doctor of ophthalmology
    D. Doctor of orthopedics

Test Your Knowledge—Answers

1. Answer: A

2. Answer: B

3. Answer: A

4. Answer: D

5. Answer: C

6. Answer: D

7. Answer: D

8. Answer: B

9. Answer: D

10. Answer: C

11. Answer: B

12. Answer: C

13. Answer: A

14. Answer: A

15. Answer: D

16. Answer: B

17. Answer: D

18. Answer: B

19. Answer: A

20. Answer: D

21. Answer: C

22. Answer: C

23. Answer: B

24. Answer: A

25. Answer: C

26. Answer: A

27. Answer: D

28. Answer: B

29. Answer: C

30. Answer: A

31. Answer: C

32. Answer: D

33. Answer: A

34. Answer: A

35. Answer: D

36. Answer: C

37. Answer: C

38. Answer: A

39. Answer: B

40. Answer: B

41. Answer: D

42. Answer: C

43. Answer: A

44. Answer: D

45. Answer: D

46. Answer: B

47. Answer: B

48. Answer: C

49. Answer: D

50. Answer: B

51. Answer: B

52. Answer: A

53. Answer: D

54. Answer: A

55. Answer: B

56. Answer: C

57. Answer: C

58. Answer: A

59. Answer: D

60. Answer: B

61. Answer: D

62. Answer: B

63. Answer: C

64. Answer: A

65. Answer: C

66. Answer: C

67. Answer: D

68. Answer: B

69. Answer: A

70. Answer: A

71. Answer: C

72. Answer: D

73. Answer: C

74. Answer: B

75. Answer: D

76. Answer: A

77. Answer: B

78. Answer: C

79. Answer: C

80. Answer: D

81. Answer: A

82. Answer: B

83. Answer: C

84. Answer: B

85. Answer: A

86. Answer: D

87. Answer: D

88. Answer: C

89. Answer: A

90. Answer: B

91. Answer: C

92. Answer: D

93. Answer: D

94. Answer: C

95. Answer: A

96. Answer: A

97. Answer: B

98. Answer: D

99. Answer: C

100. Answer: B

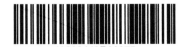

Made in the USA
Lexington, KY
01 April 2015